Bariatric Surgery - From the Non-Surgical Approach to the Post-Surgery Individual Care

Edited by Nieves Saiz-Sapena and Juan Miguel Oviedo

Published in London, United Kingdom

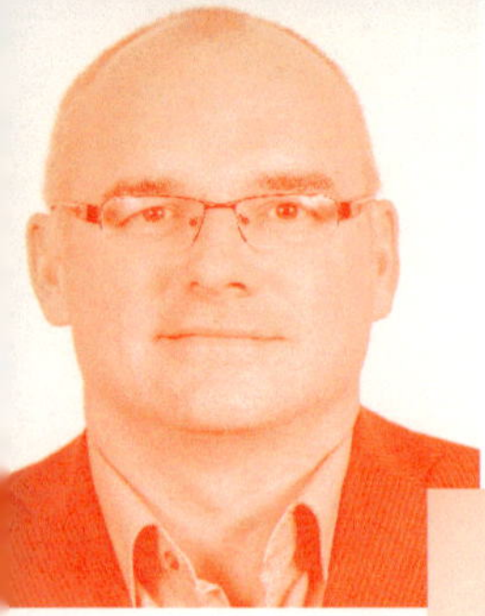
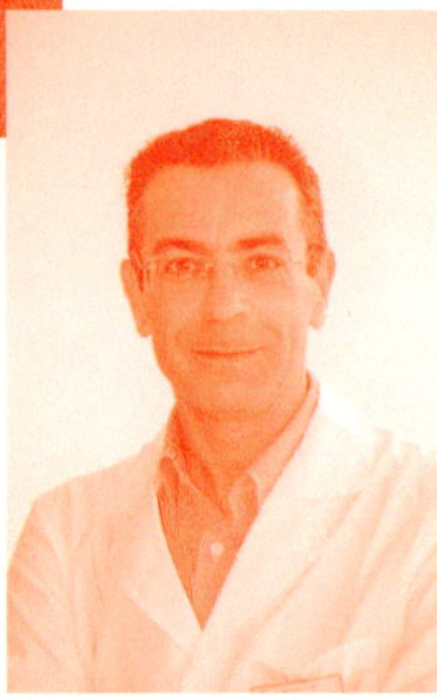
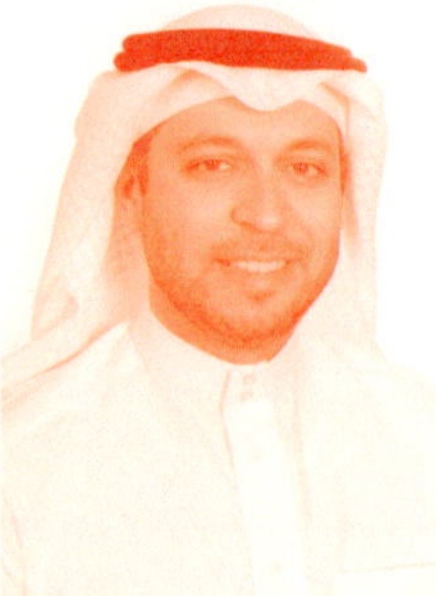
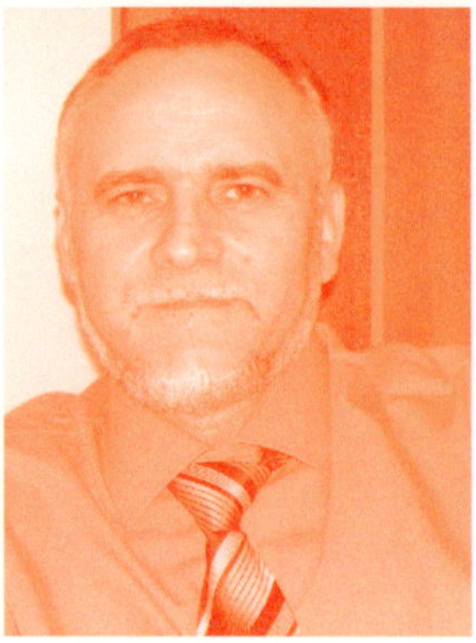
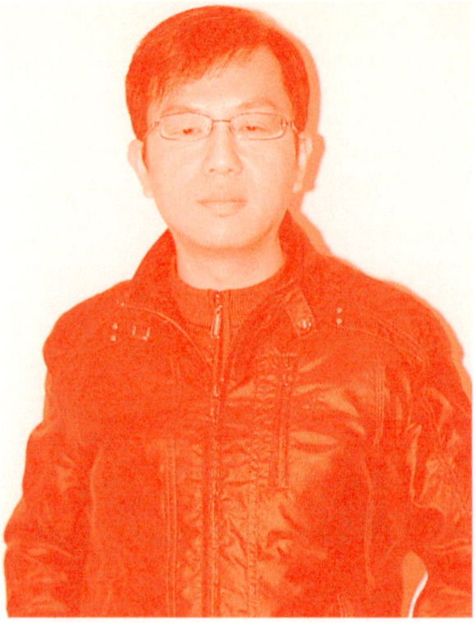
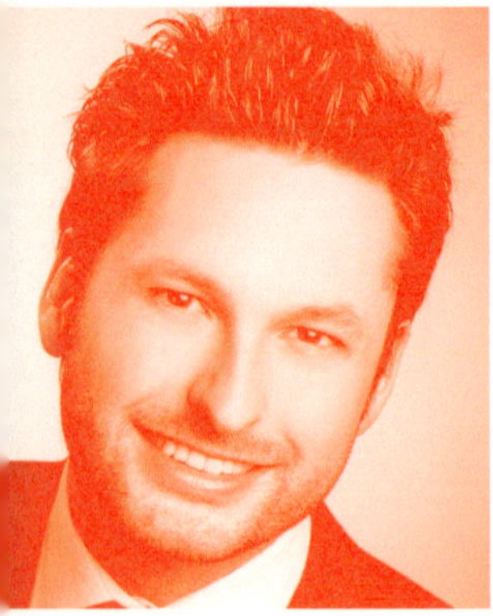
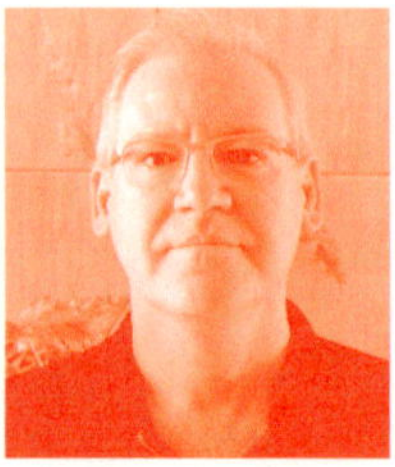

IntechOpen

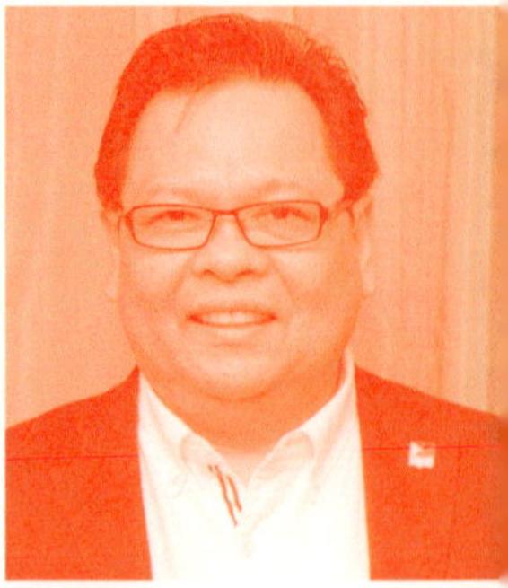
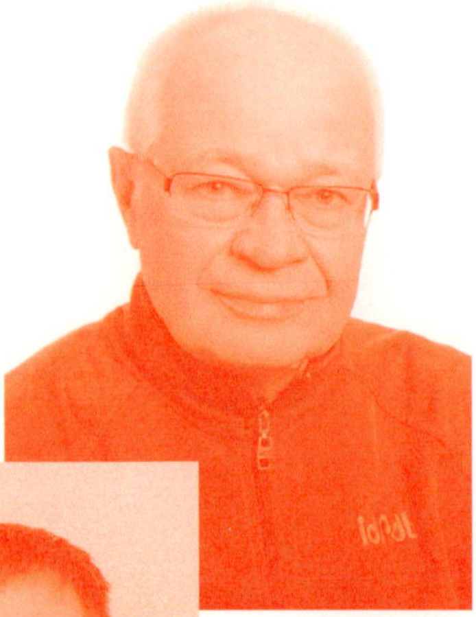
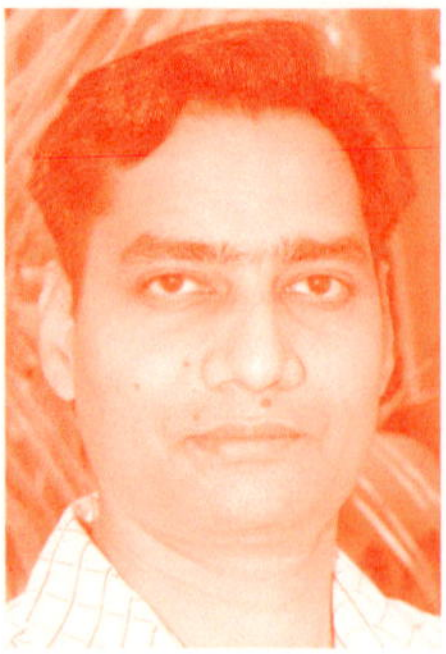
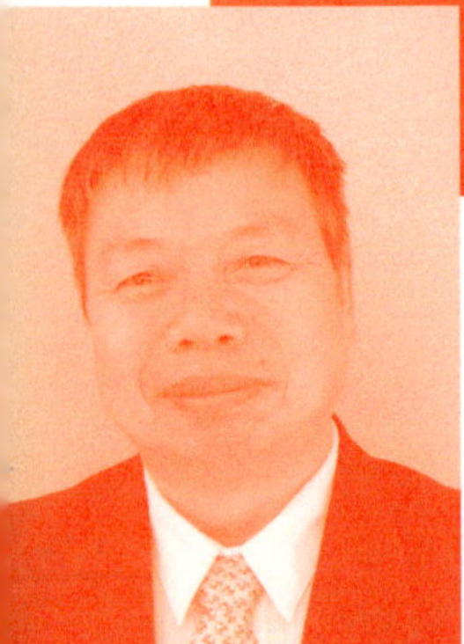
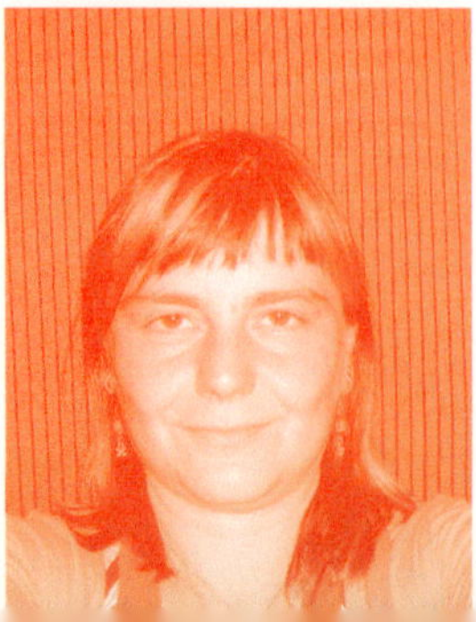
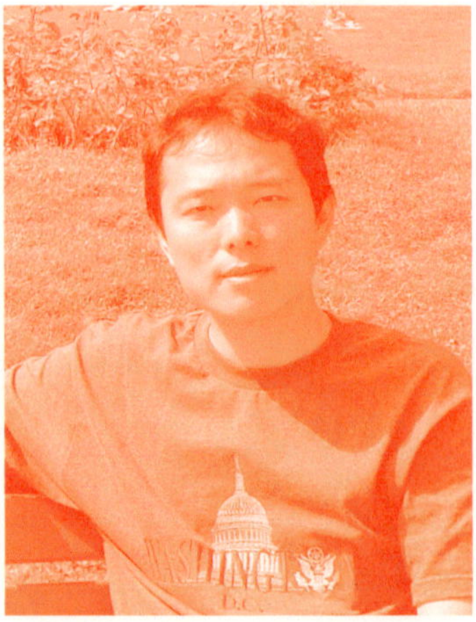

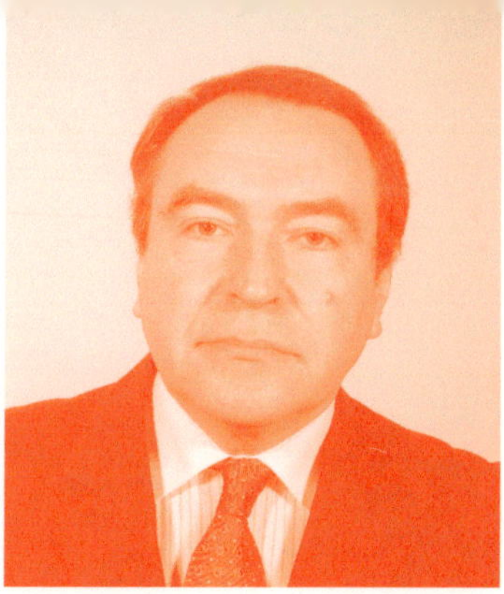
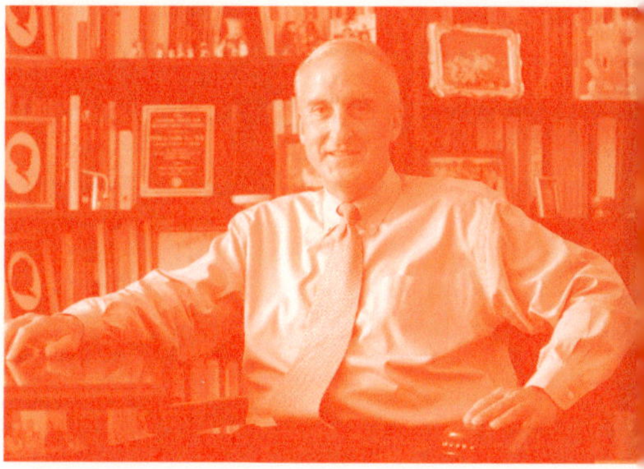
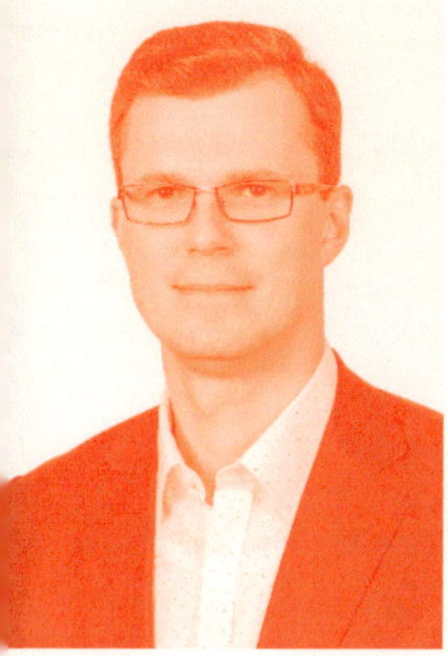
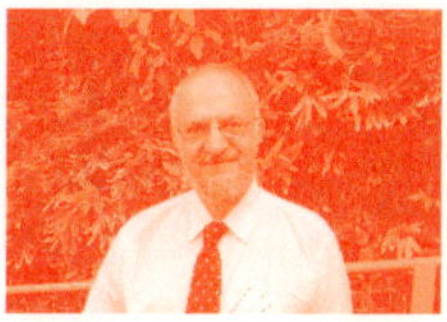
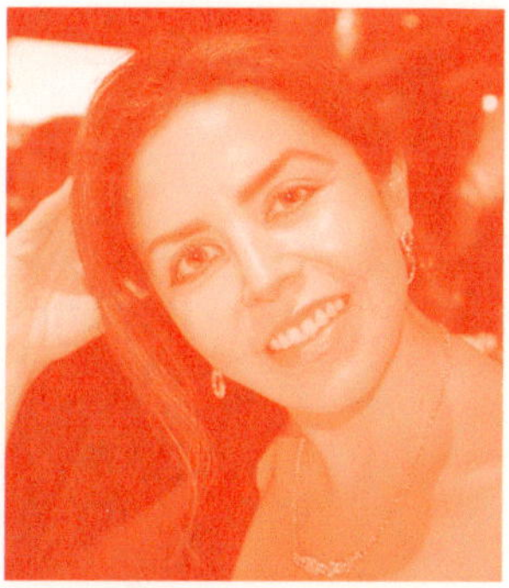

Supporting open minds since 2005

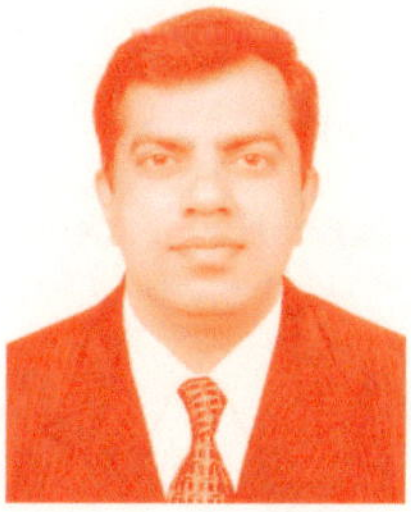
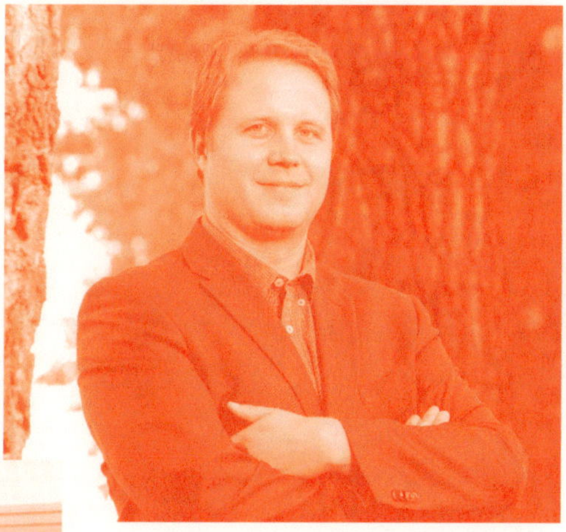
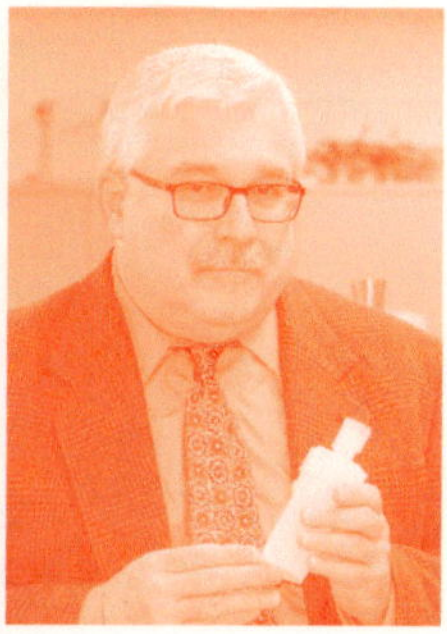
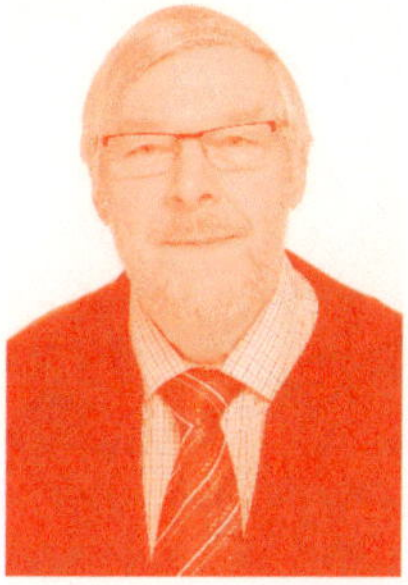
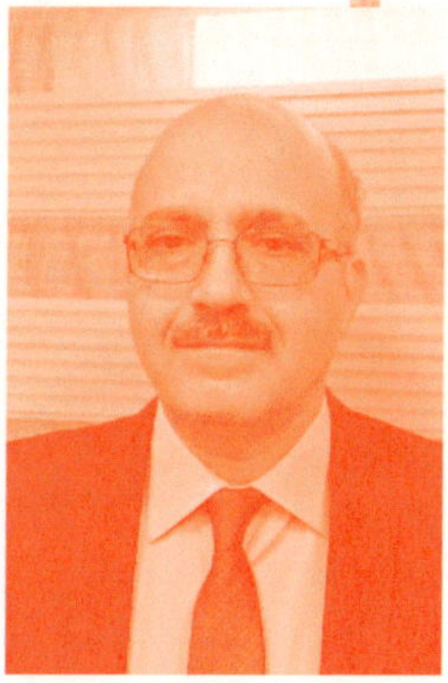
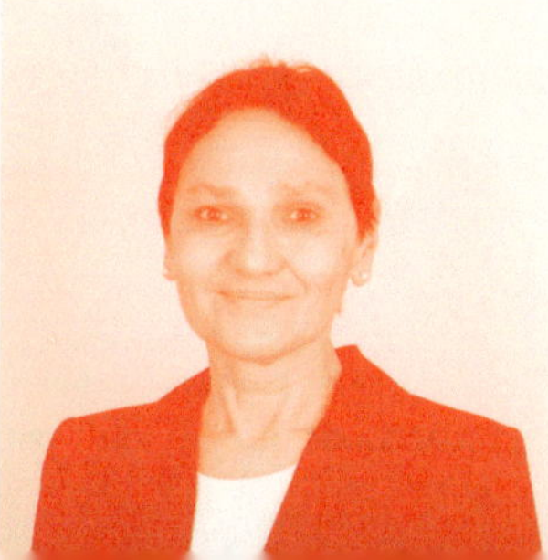
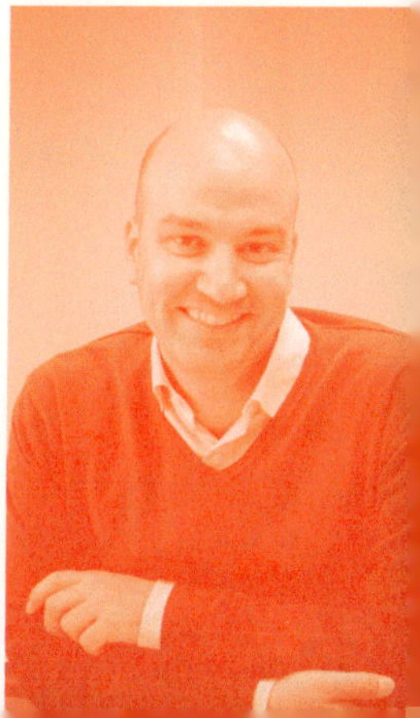

Bariatric Surgery - From the Non-Surgical Approach to the Post-Surgery Individual Care
http://dx.doi.org/10.5772/intechopen.87626
Edited by Nieves Saiz-Sapena and Juan Miguel Oviedo

Contributors
Walid El Ansari, Wahiba Elhag, Roberto Cattivelli, Anna Usubini Guerrini, Dörte Wichmann, Dietmar Stüker, Alfred Königsrainer, Rami Archid, Ulrich Schweizer, Michelle Bernadette C. Lim-Loo, Chih-Kun Huang, Valerie Chan, Kathleen Chua, Anwar Suhaimi, Brenda Saria Yuliawiratman, Veronica Mocanu, Daniel V. Timofte, Ioana Hristov, Nieves Saiz-Sapena, Juan Miguel Oviedo, Valentina Villa, Giorgia Varallo, Valentina Granese, Giada Pietrabissa, Gian Mauro Manzoni, Gianluca Castelnuovo, Enrico Molinari

First published in London, United Kingdom, 2021 by IntechOpen
IntechOpen is the global imprint of INTECHOPEN LIMITED, registered in England and Wales, registration number: 11086078, 5 Princes Gate Court, London, SW7 2QJ, United Kingdom
Printed in Croatia

British Library Cataloguing-in-Publication Data
A catalogue record for this book is available from the British Library

Additional hard and PDF copies can be obtained from orders@intechopen.com

Bariatric Surgery - From the Non-Surgical Approach to the Post-Surgery Individual Care
Edited by Nieves Saiz-Sapena and Juan Miguel Oviedo
p. cm.
Print ISBN 978-1-83968-173-8
Online ISBN 978-1-83968-174-5
eBook (PDF) ISBN 978-1-83968-175-2

For EU product safety concerns:
IN TECH d.o.o., Prolaz Marije Krucifikse Kozulić 3, 51000 Rijeka, Croatia, info@intechopen.com or visit our website at intechopen.com.

Meet the editors

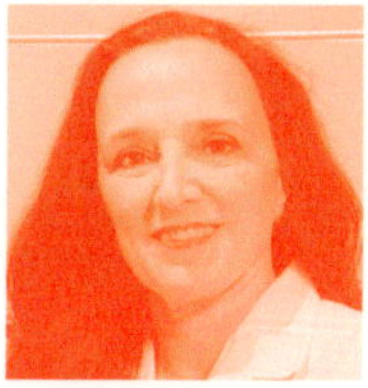

Dr. Nieves Saiz-Sapena obtained an MD from the University of Valencia, Spain, in 1988. After a short stint at the Groote Schuur Hospital, Cape Town, South Africa, she specialized in anaesthesia and intensive care and obtained a Ph.D. (cum Laude) at the University of Navarra, Spain. Dr. Saiz-Sapena has more than twenty-five years of experience in the fields of bariatric surgery, neurosurgery, hostile environments, and difficult airways. She is an active member of several scientific international societies including the International Federation for the Surgery of Obesity and Metabolic Disorders (IFSO) and the Society for Obesity and Bariatric Anaesthesia (SOBA). She is also a reviewer for national and international scientific journals. Her teaching background includes the Universidad de Navarra, Universidad de Barcelona, Universidad Cardenal Herrera-CEU, and Universidad Catolica de Valencia, both on site and online.

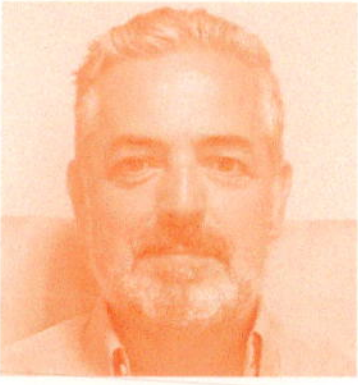

Dr. Juan Miguel Oviedo obtained an MD from the University of Sevilla, Spain, in 1992, after which he moved to Valencia, Spain, for his training as a specialist in general surgery. Since 2017, Dr. Oviedo has served as the coordinator of the Oesophagus-gastric, Bariatric, and Abdominal Wall Unit. He obtained his Ph.D. (cum laude) from the University of Valencia, Spain, in 2010, and has developed a teaching role at his hospital for the last ten years. He is also an active member of several scientific societies, including Sociedad Valenciana de Cirugia, Asociacion Española de Cirujanos (AEC), Sociedad Hispanoamericana de la Hernia (SOHAH), Sociedad Española de Cirugia de la Obesidad (SECO), and the International Federation for the Surgery of Obesity (IFSO).

Contents

Preface

The World Health Organization (WHO) defines overweight and obesity as "abnormal or excessive fat accumulation that presents a risk to health." Although obesity has been recognized as a health problem since the Middle Ages, it was not until the last century that it attracted the attention of medical departments and public health institutions. It is the cause of more than 4 million deaths per year worldwide due to not only metabolic or pathophysiological consequences but also malnutrition and lack of self-care.

Being overweight is a problem that affects half the world's population. The most severe case is the United States, where more than 68% of adults are overweight and 38% are obese. Obesity prevalence has increased globally in many countries regardless of age, sex, race, and smoking status. It has been more noticeable in the higher BMI cases (> 40 kg/m2) than in lower BMI categories (BMI < 35 kg/m2). However, causes in different countries are not fully understood.

Until the first half of the twentieth century, it was thought that persons gained weight simply because they ate too much. As such, dieting was the logical treatment to offer as well as the only treatment available. Nowadays, this thinking is outdated. Obesity is a disease that affects physical, mental, and social well-being. Multiple causes affect its development, and dieting is just one aspect of treatment.

Scientific knowledge has increased exponentially in the last 50 years. Biochemistry, pathophysiology, engineering, imaging resources, and computer science have all contributed to a better understanding of how the body works from the architectural to the molecular levels. In addition, psychology is a well-established science whose primary goals are to describe, explain, predict, and change behaviour. It helps individuals make constructive and lasting changes in their lives. Finally, social well-being cannot be fully achieved without the previous two aspects of health (physical and mental spheres).

There is a large amount of information on bariatric surgery, mainly on surgical techniques. Nowadays, the bariatric patient has to be considered as a whole, according to the WHO's definition of health. Surgery alone has a low rate of success. Bariatric treatment requires teamwork as well as dietary, social, and psychological evaluations to establish an individualized management plan that includes discharge and follow-up strategies. Besides surgical options, there are other options to offer the obese patient, including physical exercise, psychological and social support, nutrition, and pharmacological options. More recently, enhanced recovery after surgery (ERAS) protocols have highlighted the role of the anaesthesia team and perioperative care.

This book brings the reader closer to this multidisciplinary approach concept, exhibiting bariatric surgery from the non-surgical approach to post-surgery individual care, taking into account the wide range of professionals that deal with obese patients during and after treatment.

Dr. Nieves Saiz-Sapena
Department of Anaesthesiology and Intensive Care,
Consorcio Hospital General Universitario de Valencia,
Spain

Dr. Juan Miguel Oviedo
Department of Surgery – Gastro-Oesophagic Unit,
Consorcio Hospital General Universitario de Valencia,
Spain

Chapter 1

Introductory Chapter: Bariatric Surgery - Not Alone on This Long Road

Nieves Saiz-Sapena and Juan Miguel Oviedo

1. The actual burden of obesity

Obesity has become one of the leading problems worldwide and not only in first-world societies. Its prevalence rose steadily for seven decades, slowing down in the last ten years, especially in first-world countries, due to better prevention and treatment. Nevertheless, there are more overweight than underweight people in every region except sub-Saharan (but South Africa) and southeast Asian countries. Prevalence of obesity (BMI > 30%) is led by United States (38% population), Saudi Arabia (35%), Turkey, Egypt, Libya, and Canada (31–32%), and Australia (30%). In Europe, it affects 20–30% of the population, with the highest prevalence in the United Kingdom (29.5% population), followed by Hungary, Czechia, Lithuania, Greece, Bulgaria, Croatia, Spain, Ireland, Ukraine, Germany, Russia, and Poland (25.6%) [1–3].

Fat is an advancement in the evolution of the species as it allows for standing periods with no access to food and helps keep the body heat. But the convenient amount of adipose tissue has its limits, as too many fatty deposits are problematic for the skeleton, heart, pancreas, most inner organs and systems and a higher incidence of certain types of cancer [4–7]. Since the dawn of humanity, those problems have existed and are undoubtedly well-known during the roman empire decadence period [8]. It was already a problem in medieval times, but nowadays, it has reached the size of a pandemic. One of the more fundamental reasons is easy access to fast food and the consumption of high carbohydrate diets, sugar-sweetened beverages, and a more sedentary lifestyle. It is also true that access to any food is easier than ever, but some individuals cannot easily control their appetite. No one will deny the combination of availability of high caloric content food plus little caloric expenditure, but controlling their surge for food ingestion is not straightforward [9]. We all have known friends who had to be on a diet since early childhood because they were eating comparatively little, yet they kept putting on weight.

This book attempts to introduce the reader to the complex world of the treatment of obesity from a multidisciplinary point of view, from the non-surgical approach to modern surgical techniques, considering the broad spectrum of areas that may be affected in those patients.

2. The non-surgical approach

Education since childhood about the value of healthy eating is, for many, the golden bullet. But as doctors, we know that even so for a few will not be enough [10, 11]. What to do then? We cannot stand still seeing how their global health and quality of life deteriorate as they gain weight. So, modification of living style and adoption of healthy habits is taken as a real sacrifice. Then the next magic solution: bariatric surgery.

A "healthy living lifestyle" is often perceived as tedious, frustrating, tiring, too strict, not very social... but all these take us to two of the most critical issues in obesity. The first one is the psychological alteration these patients have. What was first? Did obesity lead to psychological damage? Or the other way round, is there a psychological foundation basis for obesity? In any case, psychological, dietary, and physical assessment, support, and treatment are necessary.

The second issue is the genetic propensity towards obesity. Adipose tissue works as an organ, with its own metabolic rules. And sometimes, not even the strongest-minded person can overcome it. However, the knowledge of pathophysiology has helped to individualise the treatments.

Then the next "magic solution": bariatric surgery. Preparation for such an event needs teamwork: dietitian, physiotherapist, psychologist, respiratory physician, endocrinologist, and even sometimes a personal trainer will help the patient journey to a new healthier life. Nevertheless, patients must follow a strict diet before the operation and change their minds about eating [12]. This necessary change in eating habits is, undoubtedly, the keystone for long term success. Therefore, there is an absolute need for the non-surgical approach to the bariatric patient.

3. Bariatric surgery

In the last 50 years, surgery and anaesthesia have developed exponentially compared to the previous centuries. Moreover, laparoscopy and anaesthesia-related devices and monitors have increased the safety and efficacy of surgical procedures. However, there is a 42 year time lapse from the first jejunum-ileal bypass of Kremen in 1951 [13] to the first laparoscopic bypass of Wittgrove in 1994 [14]. By then, restrictive procedures were being also introduced in bariatrics.

We all remember the adjustable gastric band in the eighties [15], which became a popular laparoscopic bariatric surgery in the nineties. Initially, patients lost weight but soon adapted to eat less and ate higher calory content [16, 17]. But, unfortunately, the band itself was also a source of many other problems like infections [18], migration [19], erosion [20] and even, on rare occasions to gastric perforation [21]. As a result, conversion to other bariatric surgical procedures has not been uncommon [22].

But with the new century also new choices came. Reducing the significant stomach curve to create a gastric sleeve with a smaller capacity was an innovative advancement. Gagner published the first experience with sleeve gastrectomy as a stand-alone procedure in 2008 [23]. It has been the solution that has helped many maintain weight within reason [24]. At this moment, it is the most common bariatric surgery type, with very low morbidity and mortality rates, making it very safe not only as a stand-alone procedure but also as the first procedure for super-obese patients. But it demands that the patient collaborates and does not do as in the gastric band: eating less but more times and with food with a high calory content [25]. The removal of the part of the stomach that segregate ghrelin helps controlling appetite, which is seen as one of the significant advantages of the procedure from the psychological point of view.

4. The post-surgical individual care

But both psychologists and nutritionists will have the most critical role at this stage. Regardless of the type of surgery, all patients need to change their habits to healthier ones, including diet, exercise, and life. In addition, family, friends, workplace, and sometimes even home need to adapt or collaborate to create a favourable and positively stimulating environment, addressed to a new life.

Changing eating habits is complicated, as homemade food needs to be increased, but sometimes there is little time. Another drawback is that some patients (most commonly those who underwent malabsorptive procedures) present iron [26] or vitamin B_{12} absorption problems [27], which might need surveillance and dietary supplementation in this respect [28].

5. Other challenges

Despite all efforts, sometimes surgery fails, and there is the weight regain. It is more common in the case of restrictive procedures, as sleeve gastrectomy. For those cases, new and ingenious surgical techniques were created [29, 30]. The basic concept is that reducing the length of the small intestine will proportionally reduce nutrient absorption [31]. Therefore, even if the patient overeats, it will not put on weight. But, sadly, the absorption of vital elements like vitamins will also be jeopardised, and these patients will need close, continuous medical surveillance and chronic dietary supplements [32–34].

Another serious challenge has been the anaesthetic and the surgical procedure themselves.

The anaesthetic itself is full of scary moments [35]. Intubating these thick necks are not that easy, especially when also arthrosis appears with age. Getting good venous and arterial lines can prove exasperating. The lung and heart functions are already at their limits, only to mention a few challenges [36, 37]. Nevertheless, the whole endocrine system is altered because of adipose tissue, with its way of behaving in metabolism terms, and we can carry on.

As far as surgery is concerned, the introduction of endoscopic techniques in the nineties made it possible to reduce surgical aggression regarding access to the anatomical structure to be treated, be it the stomach or the small intestine [38]. But with this advancement, another challenge arose. Insufflating CO_2 inside the abdominal cavity to get space for the surgical manoeuvres increases the abdominal pressure, pushing the diaphragm, thus increasing intrathoracic pressures [39]. Another challenge for the anaesthesiologist is the juggling to keep the venous return and the cardiac output within reasonable functional limits [40].

The final challenge is the patient. First, because lifestyle changes need to be maintained, the team must support the patient, but the patient must cooperate in the months following and the rest of their life. Second, the scars of the whole process will be there, showing up in the form of skin laxity, which will require, on many occasions, plastic surgery intervention, which will, in turn, will also leave its scars.

6. Conclusion

Hence, this book attempts to be a global thought on obesity and its treatment before, during and after the surgery itself, and, most importantly, in the following months and years [41]. After all, nothing is less disheartening than seeing how relentlessly some patients put back some if not all the weight lost after the bariatric surgery because long term eating habits prove to be as essential as stomach or small intestine reduction [42, 43].

Nevertheless, other essential aspects of treatment need attention before and after bariatric surgery, such as physiotherapy, micronutrient deficiencies, and psychological attention. And yet, this is not all. Many will need repeated plastic surgical procedures to recover a body image they can feel proud of, and finding a new job or a promotion in the present or a new sentimental relationship are final aspects to consider [44–47].

To conclude, obesity is much more than just a high body mass index. It entails lousy eating habits, many coming from a faulty family raising, a change in mentality about what eating must mean to keep a healthy body and understanding that others are not going to be of help through a bariatric surgery if the patient him or herself do not take an active part in the process. Bariatric surgery is a long way, but neither the patient nor the surgeon is alone. Our role as doctors in the process is tiny, and we are members of a team that will have to be around this process for long and watch for any aspect that can be improved through our help and care.

Author details

Nieves Saiz-Sapena[1*] and Juan Miguel Oviedo[2]

1 Department of Anaesthesiology, Consorcio Hospital General Universitario de Valencia, Valencia, Spain

2 Department of General Surgery, Consorcio Hospital General Universitario de Valencia, Valencia, Spain

*Address all correspondence to: nssapena@hotmail.com

References

[1] Blüher M. Obesity: Global epidemiology and pathogenesis. Nat Rev Endocrinol. 2019;15(5):288-298.

[2] National Academies of Sciences, Engineering, and Medicine; Health and Medicine Division; Food and Nutrition Board; Roundtable on Obesity Solutions. Current Status and Response to the Global Obesity Pandemic: Proceedings of a Workshop [Internet]. Callahan EA, editor. Washington (DC): National Academies Press (US); 2019. [Cited 21 May 2021]. Disponible en: http://www.ncbi.nlm.nih.gov/books/NBK544128/

[3] Prevalence of obesity among adults, BMI >= 30 (crude estimate) (%) [Internet]. [Cited 1 Agust 2021]. Disponible en: https://www.who.int/data/gho/data/indicators/indicator-details/GHO/prevalence-of-obesity-among-adults-bmi-=-30-(crude-estimate)-(-)

[4] Sung H, Siegel RL, Torre LA, Pearson-Stuttard J, Islami F, Fedewa SA, Goding Sauer A, Shuval K, Gapstur SM, Jacobs EJ, Giovannucci EL, Jemal A. Global patterns in excess body weight and the associated cancer burden. CA Cancer J Clin. 2019;69(2):88-112.

[5] Renehan AG, Soerjomataram I, Tyson M, Egger M, Zwahlen M, Coebergh JW, Buchan I. Incident cancer burden attributable to excess body mass index in 30 European countries. Int J Cancer. 2010;126(3):692-702.

[6] Kompella P, Vasquez KM. Obesity and cancer: A mechanistic overview of metabolic changes in obesity that impact genetic instability. Mol Carcinog. 2019;58(9):1531-1550.

[7] Ye P, Xi Y, Huang Z, Xu P. Linking obesity with colorectal cancer: Epidemiology and mechanistic insights. Cancers. 2020;12(6).

[8] Conti AA, Lippi D, Gensini GF. Obesity and nutritional behavior within a historical perspective. Minerva Gastroenterol Dietol. 2004;50(2):171-177.

[9] Karasu SR. Of mind and matter: Psychological dimensions in obesity. Am J Psychother. 2012;66(2):111-128.

[10] Dulloo AG, Montani J-P. Pathways from dieting to weight regain, to obesity and to the metabolic syndrome: An overview. Obes Rev Off J Int Assoc Study Obes. 2015;16 Suppl 1:1-6.

[11] Blüher M. Conservative obesity treatment – When and how? Dtsch Med Wochenschr 1946. 2015;140(1):24-8.

[12] Bettini S, Belligoli A, Fabris R, Busetto L. Diet approach before and after bariatric surgery. Rev Endocr Metab Disord. 2020;21(3):297-306.

[13] Kremen AJ, Linner JH, Nelson CH. An experimental evaluation of the nutritional importance of proximal and distal small intestine. Ann Surg 1954;140(3):439-448.

[14] Wittgrove AC, Clark GW, Tremblay LJ. Laparoscopic gastric bypass, Roux-en-Y: preliminary report of five cases. Obes Surg. noviembre de 1994;4(4):353-357.

[15] Kuzmak LI. A review of seven years' experience with silicone gastric banding. Obes Surg. 1991;1(4):403-408.

[16] Conceição E, Pinto-Bastos A, de Lourdes M, Brandão I, Teixeira C, Machado PPP. Psychological, behavioral, and weight-related aspects of patients undergoing reoperative bariatric surgery after gastric band: Comparison with primary surgery patients. Surg Obes Relat Dis Off J Am Soc Bariatr Surg. 2018;14(5):603-610.

[17] Dewberry LC, Jalivand A, Gupta R, Jenkins TM, Beamish A, Inge TH, Courcoulas A, Helmrath M, Brandt ML, Harmon CM, Chen M, Dixon JB, Zeller M, Michalsky MP. Weight loss and health status 5 years after adjustable gastric banding in adolescents. Obes Surg. 2020;30(6):2388-2394.

[18] Beh HN, Ongso YF. Simultaneous gastric and colonic erosions from gastric band and its tubing in the setting of recurrent intra-abdominal infection. J Surg Case Rep. 2019;2019(4):rjz102.

[19] Sawicka-Pierko A, Pierko J, Krawczyk M, Ładny JR, Dadan J, Hady HR. Gastric band migration to gastrointestinal lumen and possibilities of its surgical treatment. Adv Clin Exp Med Off Organ Wroclaw Med Univ. 2019;28(1):103-107.

[20] Chisholm J, Kitan N, Toouli J, Kow L. Gastric band erosion in 63 cases: Endoscopic removal and rebanding evaluated. Obes Surg. 2011;21(11):1676-1681.

[21] Sartori A, De Luca M, Clemente N, Lunardi C, Segato G, Pellicano N. Complications of laparoscopic gastric banding: Detection and treatment. Ann Ital Chir. 2017;88:206-214.

[22] Zadeh J, Le C, Ben-David K. Safety of adjustable gastric band conversion surgery: A systematic review and meta-analysis of the leak rate in 1- and 2-stage procedures. Surg Obes Relat Dis Off J Am Soc Bariatr Surg. 2020;16(3):437-444.

[23] Gagner M, Gumbs AA, Milone L, Yung E, Goldenberg L, Pomp A. Laparoscopic sleeve gastrectomy for the super-super-obese (body mass index >60 kg/m(2)). Surg Today. 2008;38(5):399-403.

[24] Stenard F, Iannelli A. Laparoscopic sleeve gastrectomy and gastroesophageal reflux. World J Gastroenterol. 2015;21(36):10348-10357.

[25] King WC, Hinerman AS, Courcoulas AP. Weight regain after bariatric surgery: A systematic literature review and comparison across studies using a large reference sample. Surg Obes Relat Dis Off J Am Soc Bariatr Surg. 2020;16(8):1133-1144.

[26] Steenackers N, Van der Schueren B, Mertens A, Lannoo M, Grauwet T, Augustijns P, Matthys C. Iron deficiency after bariatric surgery: What is the real problem? Proc Nutr Soc. 2018;77(4):445-455.

[27] Majumder S, Soriano J, Louie Cruz A, Dasanu CA. Vitamin B12 deficiency in patients undergoing bariatric surgery: Preventive strategies and key recommendations. Surg Obes Relat Dis Off J Am Soc Bariatr Surg. 2013;9(6):1013-1019.

[28] Bland CM, Quidley AM, Love BL, Yeager C, McMichael B, Bookstaver PB. Long-term pharmacotherapy considerations in the bariatric surgery patient. Am J Health-Syst Pharm AJHP Off J Am Soc Health-Syst Pharm. 2016;73(16):1230-1242.

[29] Felsenreich DM, Langer FB, Kefurt R, Panhofer P, Schermann M, Beckerhinn P, Sperker C, Prager G. Weight loss, weight regain, and conversions to Roux-en-Y gastric bypass: 10-year results of laparoscopic sleeve gastrectomy. Surg Obes Relat Dis Off J Am Soc Bariatr Surg. noviembre de 2016;12(9):1655-1662.

[30] Moon RC, Fuentes AS, Teixeira AF, Jawad MA. Conversions after sleeve gastrectomy for weight regain: To single and double anastomosis duodenal switch and gastric bypass at a single institution. Obes Surg. 2019;29(1):48-53.

[31] Bojsen-Møller KN, Jacobsen SH, Dirksen C, Jørgensen NB, Reitelseder S, Jensen J-EB, Kristiansen VB, Holst JJ, van Hall G, Madsbad S. Accelerated protein digestion and amino acid absorption

after Roux-en-Y gastric bypass. Am J Clin Nutr. 2015;102(3):600-607.

[32] Björklund P, Fändriks L. The pros and cons of gastric bypass surgery – The role of the Roux-limb. Best Pract Res Clin Gastroenterol. 2019;40-41:101638.

[33] Antoniewicz A, Kalinowski P, Kotulecka KJ, Kocoń P, Paluszkiewicz R, Remiszewski P, Zieniewicz K. Nutritional deficiencies in patients after Roux-en-Y gastric bypass and sleeve gastrectomy during 12-month follow-up. Obes Surg. 2019;29(10):3277-3284.

[34] Steenackers N, Gesquiere I, Matthys C. The relevance of dietary protein after bariatric surgery: What do we know? Curr Opin Clin Nutr Metab Care. 2018;21(1):58-63.

[35] Baumgartner P. Bariatric surgery and the gastric tube-caution for the unwary anaesthetist. Anaesth Intensive Care. 2016;44(5):644-645.

[36] Pouwels S, Buise MP, Twardowski P, Stepaniak PS, Proczko M. Obesity surgery and anesthesiology risks: A review of key concepts and related physiology. Obes Surg. 2019;29(8):2670-2677.

[37] Konrad FM, Kramer KM, Schroeder TH, Stubbig K. Anesthesia and bariatric surgery. Anaesthesist. 2011;60(7):607-616.

[38] Saunders KH, Igel LI, Saumoy M, Sharaiha RZ, Aronne LJ. Devices and endoscopic bariatric therapies for obesity. Curr Obes Rep. 2018;7(2):162-171.

[39] Eichler L, Truskowska K, Dupree A, Busch P, Goetz AE, Zöllner C. Intraoperative ventilation of morbidly obese patients guided by transpulmonary pressure. Obes Surg. 2018;28(1):122-129.

[40] Jain AK, Dutta A. Stroke volume variation as a guide to fluid administration in morbidly obese patients undergoing laparoscopic bariatric surgery. Obes Surg. 2010;20(6):709-715.

[41] Tabesh MR, Maleklou F, Ejtehadi F, Alizadeh Z. Nutrition, physical activity, and prescription of supplements in pre- and post-bariatric surgery patients: A practical guideline. Obes Surg. 2019;29(10):3385-3400.

[42] Takemoto E, Wolfe BM, Nagel CL, Pories W, Flum DR, Pomp A, Mitchell J, Boone-Heinonen J. Insurance status differences in weight loss and regain over 5 years following bariatric surgery. Int J Obes 2005. 2018;42(6):1211-20.

[43] Zarshenas N, Tapsell LC, Neale EP, Batterham M, Talbot ML. The relationship between bariatric surgery and diet quality: A systematic review. Obes Surg. 2020;30(5):1768-1792.

[44] Gilmartin J, Bath-Hextall F, Maclean J, Stanton W, Soldin M. Quality of life among adults following bariatric and body contouring surgery: A systematic review. JBI Database Syst Rev Implement Rep. 2016;14(11):240-270.

[45] Gunnarson GL, Frøyen JK, Sandbu R, Thomsen JB, Hjelmesæth J. Plastic surgery after bariatric surgery. Tidsskr Den Nor Laegeforening Tidsskr Prakt Med Ny Raekke. 2015;135(11):1044-1049.

[46] Durand-Moreau Q, Gautier A, Bécouarn G, Topart P, Rodien P, Sallé A. Employment and professional outcomes in 803 patients undergoing bariatric surgery in a French reference center for obesity. Int J Occup Environ Med. 2015;6(2):95-103.

[47] Sockalingam S, Wnuk S, Kantarovich K, Meaney C, Okrainec A, Hawa R, Cassin S. Employment outcomes one year after bariatric surgery: The role of patient and psychosocial factors. Obes Surg. 2015;25(3):514-522.

Chapter 2

Subcutaneous Adipose Stem Cells in Obesity: The Impact of Bariatric Surgery

Veronica Mocanu, Daniel V. Timofte and Ioana Hristov

Abstract

Adipocyte expansion, which involves adipose tissue-derived mesenchymal stem cells (ASCs), is a critical process with implications in the pathogenesis of metabolic syndrome and insulin resistance associated with obesity. Impaired subcutaneous adipogenesis leads to dysfunctional, hypertrophic adipocytes, chronic low-grade inflammation, and peripheric insulin resistance. Alternatively, it has also been proposed that the preservation of the functionality of subcutaneous adipocyte precursors could contribute to some obese individuals remaining metabolically healthy. Very few studies evaluated the changes in the adipogenic differentiation for human subcutaneous ASCs following bariatric surgery. Weight loss after bariatric surgery involves extensive remodeling of adipose tissue, comprising the hyperplasia-hypertrophy balance. Subcutaneous ASCs may be implicated in the variations of bariatric outcomes, through a different restoration in their proliferative and adipogenic potential. Weight loss induced by bariatric surgery correlates to the subcutaneous ASC functions and could explain the variability of metabolic improvement. Limited research data are available to the present and these data support the importance of diagnosis of subcutaneous ASCs functions as predictors of metabolic improvement after bariatric surgery.

Keywords: obesity, bariatric surgery, adipose tissue, adipose-derived stem cells

1. Introduction

Excess fat accumulation in adipose tissue causes obesity, which increases the risks of metabolic syndrome, diabetes, cardiovascular disease, and cancer. White adipose tissue (WAT) includes subcutaneous and visceral adipose tissue (SAT and VAT) with different metabolic features. SAT protects from metabolic disorders, while VAT promotes them [1].

SAT is the most important adipose tissue deposit and is characterized by its capacity to expand in reponse to surplus of energy. However, in the context of obesity, when the storage capacity of SAT is exceeded, fat is stored in other undesirable sites such as visceral depot or non-adipose organs (liver, skeletal muscle, myocardium, and pancreas). Impaired adipocyte development is associated with insulin resistance, so hypertrophic SAT is an important link with obesity-induced metabolic dysfunctions [2].

Adipocytes come from mesenchymal stem cells in the stroma of adipose tissue. These mesenchymal stem cells become preadipocytes when they lose their ability to differentiate into other mesenchymal lines and intervene in the adipocyte line. The second phase of adipogenesis is terminal differentiation, through which preadipocytes acquire the characteristics of mature adipocytes, acquiring lipid droplets and the ability to respond to hormones such as insulin. Terminal differentiation consists of a cascade of transcriptional events [3].

The number of mature adipocytes present in adipose tissue is largely determined by the ability of the limited number of preadipocytes to undergo the process of differentiation and the availability of mesenchymal cells to be differentiated into new preadipocytes when necessary [3]. Because new adipocytes are considered protective against metabolic dysfunction, it is plausible that the maladaptive adipogenesis could be involved in the pathogenesis of metabolic syndrome and insulin resistance associated with obesity [4]. In vitro studies have confirmed a decrease in the ability of adipogenic differentiation of ASCs in obese people.

The individual "set point" and the ability to expand the SAT depends on both the individual's genetic background and lifestyle. Studies have shown that obese people, metabolically healthy, have preservation of the architecture and functionality of adipose tissue. Women can recruit new fat cells in the femural or gluteal region at maturity. This ability to expand lower-body fat may reduce the abdominal subcutaneous adipocyte hypertrophy and the accumulation of ectopic visceral fat in obese women. By contrast, the reduced ability to expand SAT in lower-body region is observed in men and this is accompanied by the accumulation of fat in subcutaneous abdominal and visceral adipose tissues [5].

Adipocyte expansion, which involves adipose tissue-derived mesenchymal stem cells (ASCs), is a critical process with implications in the pathogenesis of metabolic syndrome and insulin resistance associated with obesity. Impaired subcutaneous adipogenesis leads to dysfunctional, hypertrophic adipocytes, chronic low-grade inflammation, and peripheric insulin resistance. Alternatively, it has also been proposed that the preservation of the functionality of subcutaneous adipocyte precursors could contribute to some obese individuals remaining metabolically healthy. Very few studies evaluated the changes in the adipogenic differentiation for human subcutaneous ASCs following bariatric surgery. Weight loss after bariatric surgery involves extensive adipose tissue remodeling, implicating mechanisms underlying adipose tissue plasticity, and the adipogenic potential.

2. Subcutaneous adipose stem cells

Isolation of subcutaneous human adipose stem cells

SAT consists predominantly of adipocytes, but also contains other cell populations generally referred to as the stromal vascular fraction (SVF). Studies from the 1970s first revealed that fibroblast-like cells from the cultures of the SVF [stromal vascular cultures (SVCs)] could be propagated and differentiated into mature adipocytes in vitro. These in vitro stromal vascular-derived adipocytes, named adipose stem cells (ASCs), molecularly resemble the adipocytes found in their depot of origin [6]. After the isolation and proliferation of these ASCs, they can be used for the experimental study of the molecular processes in regulating adipocyte differentiation [7].

SAT can be isolated by a minimally invasive liposuction procedure. Tissue separation studies have involved the adipose stromal and vascular compartment as the site of origin of adipose stem cells. The SVF is operationally defined as a heterogeneous mixture of cells, isolated by enzymatic dissociation and density-based separation, a procedure designed to remove the group of cells that were in the deposits around the floating adipocytes. These stromal-vascular cells represent a rich potential resource for examining a variety of ambiguities relevant to adipogenesis as well as regenerative medicine [8].

Identification of human subcutaneous adipose stem cells

Multiple cell-surface makers were demonstrated for ASC identification. The ASC immunophenotype should display the following typical marker profile for stromal cells: CD44, CD73, CD13, CD90, CD29 positive, and CD34 positive, but CD31, and CD45 negative [9]. Subcutaneous-ASC markers included CD10 and CD141 as potential cell-surface makers [10].

Compared with visceral-ASCs, subcutaneous-ASCs expressed a high level of CD90 and showed increases in proliferation, mitotic clonal expansion, and adipogenic differentiation. CD90 silencing inhibited proliferation and mitotic clonal expansion of subcutaneous-ASCs [1].

Adipogenic differentiation

Adipogenesis is the process of cell differentiation from stem cells to adipocytes. During this process, the ASCs will divide into two cells, where one cell keeps the stemness and the other cell can commit to the adipogenic lineage and become preadipocyte. The preadipocytes are fibroblast-like cells that are morphologically indistinguishable from the mesenchymal precursors but they lose their capacity to differentiate into other cell types (osteocytes, chondrocytes, myocytes, etc. The preadipocyte can terminal differentiate and acquire the characteristics of mature adipocytes, including lipid synthesis, insulin sensitivity, and the secretion of adipocyte-specific proteins. The terminally-differentiated adipocytes are characterized by a large unilocular lipid droplet and their main function is energy storage [11].

Adipogenesis is a well-orchestrated process that requires sequential activation of numerous transcription factors, including the CCAAT gene family/enhancer-binding protector (C/EBP) and peroxisomal proliferator-activated receptor-γ (PPAR-γ) [12]. The molecular mechanisms of adipogenesis involve stimulators and inhibitors. Adipogenic stimulators are represented by peroxisome proliferator-activated γ receptor (PPAR γ), insulin-like growth factor I (IGF-1), macrophage colony-stimulating factor, fatty acids, prostaglandins, and glucocorticoids. The inhibitors are Wnt, transforming growth factor-β (TGF-β), inflammatory cytokines, and growth hormone. Adipogenesis could be also influenced by age, gender, adipose depot, and lifestyle [13].

In vitro studies showed that mRNA expression level of CD10 of subcutaneous-ASCs increased after adipogenic stimuli, and this increase positively correlated with those of adipogenic markers, PPARG and aP2. In contrast, the CD200 level decreased after adipogenesis was initiated and exhibited a negative correlation with adipogenic markers [10].

Microenvironment of ASCs

Stem cells are found in a specialized environment, a niche, which controls many aspects of cell behavior - activity, proliferation, and differentiation The microenvironment of the subcutaneous stem cell (niche) refers to a specific location în which the adult subcutaneous cells reside and interact with ASCs and other cells or substrates. The surrounding microenvironment of ASCs provides signals that keep ASCs quiescent or promote either proliferation or differentiation. However, the niche function is to prevent ASC proliferation or differentiation. Several important factors regulate ASCs' characteristics within the niche, including cell–cell and cell-extracellular matrix (ECM) relationships, growth factors, oxygen tension, and cytokine signals [11].

3. Subcutaneous ASCs differentiation in obesity

In obese patients, adipose tissue expands by differentiating preadipocytes into adipocytes (adipogenesis) and/or hypertrophy of existing adipocytes. Adipocytes hyperplasia is the alternative optimal process for sustaining the high demand for lipid storage, through the activation of multipotent stem cells, leading to the generation of new mature adipose cells, but it has a limited and individualized capacity [14, 15].

The low adipogenic capacity of subcutaneous ASCs may result in a dysfunctional tissue, because it leads to adipocyte hypertrophy, causing the accumulation of inflammatory macrophages; insulin resistance; and also the accumulation of ectopic fats in the liver, muscles, kidneys, and pancreas [16–21].

The subcutaneous ASC functions are altered in obese patients. The literature review on the relationship between obesity and adipogenic differentiation capacity of mesenchymal stem cells originating in subcutaneous adipose tissue obtained from pre-surgical obese patients are shown in **Table 1**.

Several studies found that lipid accumulation in hypertrophic subcutaneous adipocytes evaluates the expansion capacity of the pre-adipogenic mesenchymal cell line and lipid overloaded adipocytes are associated with a poor metabolic profile for obese patients [28–30]. The subcutaneous adipose tissue represents 90% of total fat mass, it has the potential to greatly affect systemic insulin resistance via adipokine secretion in obese persons [31].

The obese population is known to be at high risk for cardio-metabolic diseases. Insulin resistance evaluation by HOMA-IR is considered as a good cardiovascular

Study (authors, year)	Results regarding adipogenesis	Particularities (group/study)
De Girolamo et al., 2013 [22]	Reduced ASCs proliferation and slightly reduced differentiation in obese vs. non-obese patients;	Human subcutaneous ASCs from bariatric obese patients (BMI > 35 kg/m^2, N = 8) vs. non-obese (BMI < 30 kg/m^2, N = 7);
Frazier et al., 2013 [23]	Reduced ASCs proliferation in overweight patients, without significant effect on adipogenic differentiation;	Human lipo-aspirate isolated ASCs overweight patients (BMI > 25 kg/m^2, N = 6) vs. normal weight patients (BMI < 25 kg/m^2, N = 8);
Hristov et al., 2019 [24]	Reduced adipogenic potential. Negative correlations with HOMA-IR and leptin/adiponectin ratio.	Human subcutaneous ASCs from bariatric obese women (N = 20; BMI = 45 ± 10 kg/m^2) and normal weight women (N = 7; BMI = 24.5 ± 2.5 kg/m^2);
Muir et al., 2016 [25]	No difference in preadipocyte frequency between DM and NDM subjects was observed in SAT.	Human subcutaneous ASCs from bariatric obese patients: diabetic, DM (BMI =47 kg/m^2; N = 34) and non-diabetic, NDM (BMI =47 kg/m^2; N = 48)
Oliva-Olivera et al., 2017 [26]	Reduced adipogenic gene expression in overweight patients;	Human subcutaneous ASCs; overweight patients (BMI > 25 kg/m^2, N = 20) vs. normal weight patients (BMI < 25 kg/m^2, N = 40);
Pachón-Peña et al., 2016 [27]	Reduced proliferation and migration capacity, and reduced adipogenic differentiation potential independent of oxygen tension;	Human lipo-aspirate isolated ASCs from obese patients (N = 8; BMI: 35 ± kg/m^2) and normal weight patients (N = 8; BMI = 23 ± 1 kg/m^2);

Table 1.
Relationship between subcutaneous ASCs and obesity in pre-surgical patients.

risk predictor [32], is also demonstrated as a valuable criterion for identifying obese individuals with a higher mortality risk by Hinnouho et al. [33].

Insulin resistance and its cardio-metabolic consequences are closely associated with disturbances of fat metabolism, as it was demonstrated that exceeding the subcutaneous adipose tissues storage capacity results in fatty acid infiltration of insulin target tissues like the skeletal muscle and the liver [34], a phenomenon known as lipotoxicity that is intimately related to the development of insulin resistance.

The estimated prevalence of obese patients without metabolic syndrome criteria in a recent meta-analysis is 35% of the obese patients [35], so it becomes important to better understand the particularities of adiposity expansion in these obese patients that do not develop insulin-resistance or associated metabolic disturbances.

Effects of hyperglycemia and oxidative stress on subcutaneous ASC adipogenesis

Diabetes impairs the angiogenic potential of adipose-derived stem cells by selectively depleting cellular subpopulations. Studying adipogenic potential of adipose tissue-derived from diabetic type 1 or type 2 mice, Rennert et al. [36] observed depletion of putative ASCs (CD45-/CD31-/CD34+ cells) within the diabetic SVF, which was consistent with the signaling dysfunction seen in this environment.

Recent studies have shown the widespread downregulation of mesenchymal stem cell markers in the SAT of diabetic rats. ASCs derived from obese mice [37] and Zucker diabetic fatty rats [38] exhibited a reduced capability for adipogenic differentiation associated with a decreased expression of related genes insulin receptor substrate 1 (IRS1), insulin receptor substrate 2 (IRS2), and adipocyte fatty acid-binding protein (aP2 or FABP4) compared with mouse control ASCs.

The oxidative stress generated by hyperglycemia has deleterious effects on proliferation, survival, homing, and angiogenic capacity of ASCs derived from the stromal vascular fraction [11, 39, 40]. Hyperglycemia up-regulates reactive oxygen species (ROS) production, suppresses the nitric oxide (NO) synthesis pathway, thereby may impair the regenerative function of ASCs. Impaired adipogenesis and IR were associated with increased 4-HNE, increased 8-hydroxy-2-deoxyguanosine (8-OHdG), increased cholesterol oxidation-derived oxysterols [41]. Also, it was demonstrated that the heme oxygenase-1 inhibited proliferation and differentiation of preadipocytes at the onset of obesity via reactive oxygen species-dependent activation of Akt/PKB (protein kinase B) in obese mouse models [42].

The mechanism of decreased number of stem cells in murine diabetic adipose tissue may involve the activation of hyaluronan synthases in intracellular membrane compartments [43]. The study by Han et al. [44] showed that extended extracellular hyaluronan matrices were found around adipocytes in obese mice. The matrix was infiltrated with macrophages, which would otherwise accumulate because adipocytes would continue to synthesize and extrude hyaluronan indefinitely in response to sustained hyperglycemia. The stem cells that divide into hyperglycemia (> 2.5 times normal) are heading for pathological adipogenesis in response to glucose stress and that subsequent cell divisions along this pathway could contribute to the expanded population of fat cells in adipose tissue in diabetes.

Effects of pro-inflammatory signals on subcutaneous ASC adipogenesis

Obesity is characterized by the accumulation of diverse immune cells in both the subcutaneous and visceral expanding fat depots, even though macrophage infiltration appears to be more prominent in the latter [45]. The presence of macrophages in the human SAT is causally related to impaired ASCs differentiation, which in turn is associated with systemic IR. A negative correlation between SAT adipogenesis, but not VAT, and systemic IR was observed [46]. Moreover, lipid-laden adipocytes produce increased levels of cytokines such as Interleukin 6 (IL-6), IL-1β, IL-8, TNF-α, and monocyte chemoattractant protein-1 (MCP-1), which can inhibit preadipocyte differentiation [41].

To investigate the inflammatory state in diabetes, the levels of IL1β, IL-6, and TNFα were measured. Numerous studies have shown these cytokines reduce adipogenesis. In patients with diabetes, IL-1β has been shown to induce insulin resistance (IR) in adipocytes by reducing IRS-1 regulation. Also, decreased IRS-1 expression has been reported to inhibit adipogenesis by decreasing CEBPα and PPARγ. Finally, the expression of SIRT1 is downregulated compared to that of healthy cells, this finding is consistent with other studies showing that inhibition of this enzyme increases senescence and reduces the proliferation of MSCs, losing their adipogenic potential [21].

Recent studies revealed that IL-6 may be a good marker of subcutaneous adipose tissue inflammation and it is inversely related to adipogenic capacity. Subcutaneous ASCs derived from insulin-resistance obese individuals exhibited a lower pro-adipogenic and higher anti-adipogenic gene expression profile This diminished adipogenic potential of ASCs may be a consequence of a preponderance of large adipocytes, prone to forming inflammatory foci. Markers of oxidative stress were also elevated in the IR state. Thus the related scenario of inflammation and oxidative stress is a likely mediator of increased IL-6 secretion in this depot [47].

4. Bariatric surgery impact on subcutaneous ASCs differentiation

Bariatric surgery is widely acknowledged as the most effective treatment for obesity (Frikke-Schmidt, O'Rourke et al. 2016). The most obvious effect of bariatric surgery is a loss of up to half of the total adipose tissue mass within the first year after surgery along with improvements in systemic metabolism.

Weight loss after bariatric surgery involves extensive remodeling of adipose tissue, comprising the hyperplasia-hypertrophy balance. The bariatric intervention has variable results, with up to 35% of patients achieving suboptimal weight loss [48]. ASC adipogenic potential correlates of metabolic disease and therapeutic responses are poorly defined. Very few published data that correlate changes in weight loss induced by bariatric surgery and preadipocyte functions (**Table 2**).

In obesity, subcutaneous ASCs have abnormal functions in terms of angiogenic differentiation, proliferation, migration, viability, and an altered and inflammatory transcriptome [51, 52]. Weight loss partially rescues some of the aforementioned features.

An important improvement in glycemia is seen in obese patients with diabetes who undergo bariatric surgery, even before clinically significant weight loss occurs. A decrease of 50% in HOMA-IR is seen within 1 week following surgery [53]. Partial or total remission rates in type 2 diabetes as high as 80–90% have been observed to occur following bariatric surgery [54, 55].

Few studies have successfully measured local inflammation within subcutaneous adipose tissues after surgery in human studies. However, these limited findings do indicate that adipose tissue infiltration decreases [56]. A shift in the distribution of the remaining macrophages was also observed, including two features: 1) disappearance of CLS, and 2) macrophages located near blood vessels [56]. The studies that investigated the impact of bariatric surgery on mRNA expression of total macrophage cell marker CD68 in abdominal subcutaneous AT and showed a significant CD68 mRNA expression levels were significantly decreased 12 and 24 months after bariatric surgery but not after 6 months [57–60].

Studies in rodents suggest that although subcutaneous ASCs derived from mice with partial weight loss present an improved proliferative ability, lipid accumulation was lower than in control differentiated ASCs. The inefficient lipid storage could indicate that after weight loss, ASCs do not recover the ability to differentiate

Study (authors, year)	Results regarding adipogenesis	Particularities (lot/study)
Mitterberger et al., 2014 [49]	Higher adipogenic differentiation rates for ASCs from former obese patients after significant lifestyle intervention weight loss;	Human subcutaneous ASCs from obese, OD (N = 4, BMI ≥ 30 kg/m^2), long-term calorically restricted initially obese, CRD (N = 4, former BMI ≥ 30 kg/m^2, current BMI ≤ 30) and normal weight, NWD (N = 4, BMI 19–25 kg/m^2).
Muir et al., 2017 [48]	A direct correlation between pre-bariatric subcutaneous ASC frequency and weight loss (12 month-%TWL);	Human subcutaneous ASCs from bariatric obese patients: diabetic, DM (BMI =46 kg/m2; N = 37); prediabetic PRE (BMI =48 kg/m^2; N = 26), and non-diabetic, NDM (BMI =46 kg/m^2; N = 32)
Silva et al., 2015 [50]	The ASCs from post-bariatric surgery ex-obese patients showed the highest levels of lipid accumulation whereas those from the obese women had the lowest levels. ASC behavior is altered in the subcutaneous adipose tissue of morbidly obese women; these changes are not completely restored after bariatric surgery-induced weight loss.	Human subcutaneous ASCs from bariatric obese women (N = 12, BMI = 46.2 ± 5.1 kg/m^2) and post bariatric surgery ex-obese women (N = 7, initial BMI = 47.8 ± 1.3 kg/m^2) and normal-weight women (N = 6, BMI = 27.5 ± 0.5 kg/m^2; final BMI = 28.1 ± 1.1 kg/m^2)

Table 2.
Relationship between subcutaneous ASCs and weight loss induced by surgical interventions.

to the adipocyte lineage. These studies indicate that reduced energy intake might create a protective environment [37].

Mitterberger et al. [49] provided evidence suggesting that long-term caloric restriction-induced by diet and bariatric surgery reduced DNA-damage, improved viability, extended replicative lifespan, and reduced adipogenic differentiation potential of subcutaneous ASCs in formerly obese women.

Muir et al. [48] observed a relationship between pre-surgical subcutaneous ASCs frequency and surgery-induced weight loss only in women, suggesting different sex-specific mechanisms of tissue remodeling associated with bariatric surgery weight loss responses. [48]. These findings indicate that the diagnosis of ASCs functions pre-bariatric surgery could predict the level of metabolic changes following bariatric surgery. This data would allow specialists to establish some criteria for the selection of obese patients with metabolic comorbidities for whom bariatric surgery would have the greatest benefit.

5. Diagnosis of abdominal subcutaneous ASC differentiation as a predictor of weight loss and metabolic outcome in bariatric patients

Large evidence indicates that enlargement of adipocytes in obesity is associated with low-grade chronic inflammation which further leads to abnormal adipokine release and impaired glucose metabolism [61]. In obese patients with associated diabetes mellitus, VAT contains larger adipocytes and fewer preadipocytes as compared to SAT [62]. However, studies that examined the relationship between generalized and regional adiposity and insulin sensitivity in type 2 diabetic patients concluded that upper-body SAT (abdominal) plays a major role in obesity-related insulin resistance in comparison to visceral or retroperitoneal fat. These results suggest that upper-body SAT had a stronger correlation with insulin sensitivity than VAT among type 2 diabetic men [16].

Studying the response to overfeeding in upper- and lower-body SAT, Tchoukalova et al. [63] reported the hypertrophy of upper-body (abdominal) adipocyte and hyperplasia of lower-body (gluteofemoral) adipocyte to over-feeding in healthy men. In morbidly obese women with normal plasma glucose concentrations, mean adipocyte volume was larger in VAT than that in SAT, but these two depots did not differ in the proportion of small adipocytes. The ability of metabolically healthy obese to expand lower-body fat is a protective mechanism involving a hyperplastic response to energy overload. High rates of adipogenesis were associated with a smaller size of abdominal subcutaneous adipocytes, lower waist-to-hip ratio, and more favorable metabolic profile [63].

In bariatric patients, the adipocyte size and the preadipocyte content were assessed in SAT (abdominal) and VAT (greater omentum) by Muir et al. [25]. They observed modest correlations between adipocyte size and weight loss only in VAT. Independently of adipocyte size, the surgery-induced weight loss (12 month-%TWL) was direct correlated with pre-surgical preadipocyte frequency only in female subjects and this correlation was more robust in SAT than VAT.

Recently, CT-derived radiodensity measurement has been validated against ex-vivo adipose tissue samples for the assessment of tissue lipid. In morbidly obese patients, lower CT-derived adipose tissue radiodensity (corresponding to higher lipid content) in abdominal fat depots was associated with metabolic disorders [64, 65]. The post-surgery increase in abdominal SAT and VAT radiodensities reflecting decreased lipid content, increased tissue blood flow rate, and diminishing adipose inflammation was associated with a favorable metabolic state.

There is a growing body of evidence to suggest that studying the abdominal subcutaneous ASCs differentiation using biopsies or adipose CT radiodensity is important to understand the tissue responses to weight loss. The diagnosis of the adipogenic potential of abdominal subcutaneous ASC could predict the weight-loss and metabolic outcome in obese patients following bariatric surgery.

6. Conclusions

Subcutaneous ASCs may be implicated in the variations of bariatric outcomes, through a different restoration in their proliferative and adipogenic potential. Weight loss induced by bariatric surgery correlates to the subcutaneous ASC functions and could explain the variability of metabolic improvement. Limited research data are available to the present and these data support the importance of diagnosis of subcutaneous ASCs functions as predictors of metabolic improvement after bariatric surgery.

Author details

Veronica Mocanu[1], Daniel V. Timofte[2*] and Ioana Hristov[1]

1 Department of MorphoFunctional Sciences, Grigore T. Popa University of Medicine and Pharmacy, Iasi, Romania,

2 Department of Surgery, Grigore T. Popa University of Medicine and Pharmacy, Iasi, Romania

*Address all correspondence to: daniel.timofte@umfiasi.ro; dantimofte@yahoo.com

References

[1] Pan Z, Zhou Z, Zhang H, Zhao H, Song P, Wang D, et al. CD90 serves as differential modulator of subcutaneous and visceral adipose-derived stem cells by regulating AKT activation that influences adipose tissue and metabolic homeostasis. Stem Cell Res Ther. 2019;10(1):355.

[2] Kim SM, Lun M, Wang M, Senyo SE, Guillermier C, Patwari P, et al. Loss of white adipose hyperplastic potential is associated with enhanced susceptibility to insulin resistance. Cell Metab. 2014;20(6):1049-1058.

[3] Ali AT, Hochfeld WE, Myburgh R, Pepper MS. Adipocyte and adipogenesis. Eur J Cell Biol. 2013;92(6-7):229-236.

[4] Longo M, Zatterale F, Naderi J, Parrillo L, Formisano P, Raciti GA, et al. Adipose Tissue Dysfunction as Determinant of Obesity-Associated Metabolic Complications. Int J Mol Sci. 2019;20(9).

[5] Gustafson B, Hedjazifar S, Gogg S, Hammarstedt A, Smith U. Insulin resistance and impaired adipogenesis. Trends Endocrinol Metab. 2015;26(4):193-200.

[6] Wang QA, Scherer PE, Gupta RK. Improved methodologies for the study of adipose biology: insights gained and opportunities ahead. J Lipid Res. 2014;55(4):605-624.

[7] Russo V, Yu C, Belliveau P, Hamilton A, Flynn LE. Comparison of human adipose-derived stem cells isolated from subcutaneous, omental, and intrathoracic adipose tissue depots for regenerative applications. Stem Cells Transl Med. 2013;3(2):206-217.

[8] Karina K, Rosliana I, Rosadi I, Schwartz R, Sobariah S, Afini I, et al. Safety of Technique and Procedure of Stromal Vascular Fraction Therapy: From Liposuction to Cell Administration. Scientifica (Cairo). 2020;2020:2863624.

[9] Gentile P, Calabrese C, De Angelis B, Pizzicannella J, Kothari A, Garcovich S. Impact of the Different Preparation Methods to Obtain Human Adipose-Derived Stromal Vascular Fraction Cells (AD-SVFs) and Human Adipose-Derived Mesenchymal Stem Cells (AD-MSCs): Enzymatic Digestion Versus Mechanical Centrifugation. Int J Mol Sci. 2019;20(21).

[10] Ong WK, Tan CS, Chan KL, Goesantoso GG, Chan XH, Chan E, et al. Identification of specific cell-surface markers of adipose-derived stem cells from subcutaneous and visceral fat depots. Stem Cell Reports. 2014;2(2):171-179.

[11] Karina K, Rosadi I, Pawitan JA. Adipose-derived stem cells and their microenvironment (Niche) in type 2 diabetes mellitus. Stem Cell Investigation. 2019;7:2-.

[12] Chang E, Kim CY. Natural Products and Obesity: A Focus on the Regulation of Mitotic Clonal Expansion during Adipogenesis. Molecules. 2019;24(6).

[13] Tang QQ, Lane MD. Adipogenesis: from stem cell to adipocyte. Annu Rev Biochem. 2012;81:715-736.

[14] Andersson DP, Eriksson Hogling D, Thorell A, Toft E, Qvisth V, Naslund E, et al. Changes in subcutaneous fat cell volume and insulin sensitivity after weight loss. Diabetes Care. 2014;37(7):1831-1836.

[15] Lonn M, Mehlig K, Bengtsson C, Lissner L. Adipocyte size predicts incidence of type 2 diabetes in women. FASEB J. 2010;24(1):326-331.

[16] Patel P, Abate N. Body fat distribution and insulin resistance. Nutrients. 2013;5(6):2019-2027.

[17] Rosen ED, Spiegelman BM. Molecular regulation of adipogenesis. Annu Rev Cell Dev Biol. 2000;16:145-171.

[18] Butcovan D, Oboroceanu T, Cimpeanu C, Mironescu A, Haliga RE, Pinzariu AC, et al. The Involvement of Epicardial Adiposity and Inflammation in Postoperatory Atrial Fibrilation - Immunohistochemical Qualitative and Quantitative Assessment. REVCHIM(Bucharest). 2017;68(4):886-9.

[19] Aursulesei V, Bulughiana S, Stoica B, Anisie E. Circulating Chemerin, Oxidative Stress, Inflammation and Insulin Resistance in Morbid Obesity Rev Chim (Bucharest). 2017; 68, No(5):1014-8.

[20] Mihai BM, Petris AO, Ungureanu DA, Lacatusu CM. Insulin resistance and adipokine levels correlate with early atherosclerosis - a study in prediabetic patients. Open Med (Wars). 2015;10(1):14-24.

[21] Barbagallo I, Li Volti G, Galvano F, Tettamanti G, Pluchinotta FR, Bergante S, et al. Diabetic human adipose tissue-derived mesenchymal stem cells fail to differentiate in functional adipocytes. Exp Biol Med (Maywood). 2017;242(10):1079-1085.

[22] De Girolamo L, Stanco D, Salvatori L, Coroniti G, Arrigoni E, Silecchia G, et al. Stemness and osteogenic and adipogenic potential are differently impaired in subcutaneous and visceral adipose derived stem cells (ASCs) isolated from obese donors. Int J Immunopathol Pharmacol. 2013;26(1 Suppl):11-21.

[23] Frazier TP, Gimble JM, Devay JW, Tucker HA, Chiu ES, Rowan BG. Body mass index affects proliferation and osteogenic differentiation of human subcutaneous adipose tissue-derived stem cells. BMC Cell Biol. 2013;14:34.

[24] Hristov I, Mocanu V, Zugun-Eloae F, Labusca L, Cretu-Silivestru I, Oboroceanu T, et al. Association of intracellular lipid accumulation in subcutaneous adipocyte precursors and plasma adipokines in bariatric surgery candidates. Lipids Health Dis. 2019;18(1):141.

[25] Muir LA, Neeley CK, Meyer KA, Baker NA, Brosius AM, Washabaugh AR, et al. Adipose tissue fibrosis, hypertrophy, and hyperplasia: Correlations with diabetes in human obesity. Obesity (Silver Spring). 2016;24(3):597-605.

[26] Oliva-Olivera W, Coin-Araguez L, Lhamyani S, Clemente-Postigo M, Torres JA, Bernal-Lopez MR, et al. Adipogenic Impairment of Adipose Tissue-Derived Mesenchymal Stem Cells in Subjects With Metabolic Syndrome: Possible Protective Role of FGF2. J Clin Endocrinol Metab. 2017;102(2):478-487.

[27] Pachon-Pena G, Serena C, Ejarque M, Petriz J, Duran X, Oliva-Olivera W, et al. Obesity Determines the Immunophenotypic Profile and Functional Characteristics of Human Mesenchymal Stem Cells From Adipose Tissue. Stem Cells Transl Med. 2016;5(4):464-475.

[28] Isakson P, Hammarstedt A, Gustafson B, Smith U. Impaired preadipocyte differentiation in human abdominal obesity: role of Wnt, tumor necrosis factor-alpha, and inflammation. Diabetes. 2009;58(7):1550-1557.

[29] McLaughlin T, Deng A, Yee G, Lamendola C, Reaven G, Tsao PS, et al. Inflammation in subcutaneous adipose

tissue: relationship to adipose cell size. Diabetologia. 2010;53(2):369-377.

[30] Vidal-Puig A. Adipose tissue expandability, lipotoxicity and the metabolic syndrome. Endocrinol Nutr. 2013;60 Suppl 1:39-43.

[31] Jeffery E, Church CD, Holtrup B, Colman L, Rodeheffer MS. Rapid depot-specific activation of adipocyte precursor cells at the onset of obesity. Nat Cell Biol. 2015;17(4):376-385.

[32] Meigs JB, Wilson PW, Fox CS, Vasan RS, Nathan DM, Sullivan LM, et al. Body mass index, metabolic syndrome, and risk of type 2 diabetes or cardiovascular disease. J Clin Endocrinol Metab. 2006;91(8):2906-2912.

[33] Hinnouho GM, Czernichow S, Dugravot A, Batty GD, Kivimaki M, Singh-Manoux A. Metabolically healthy obesity and risk of mortality: does the definition of metabolic health matter? Diabetes Care. 2013;36(8):2294-2300.

[34] Virtue S, Vidal-Puig A. It's not how fat you are, it's what you do with it that counts. PLoS Biol. 2008;6(9):e237.

[35] Lin H, Zhang L, Zheng R, Zheng Y. The prevalence, metabolic risk and effects of lifestyle intervention for metabolically healthy obesity: a systematic review and meta-analysis: A PRISMA-compliant article. Medicine (Baltimore). 2017;96(47):e8838.

[36] Rennert RC, Sorkin M, Januszyk M, Duscher D, Kosaraju R, Chung MT, et al. Diabetes impairs the angiogenic potential of adipose-derived stem cells by selectively depleting cellular subpopulations. Stem Cell Res Ther. 2014;5(3):79.

[37] Perez LM, Suarez J, Bernal A, de Lucas B, San Martin N, Galvez BG. Obesity-driven alterations in adipose-derived stem cells are partially restored by weight loss. Obesity (Silver Spring). 2016;24(3):661-669.

[38] Ferrer-Lorente R, Bejar MT, Tous M, Vilahur G, Badimon L. Systems biology approach to identify alterations in the stem cell reservoir of subcutaneous adipose tissue in a rat model of diabetes: effects on differentiation potential and function. Diabetologia. 2014;57(1):246-256.

[39] Saki N, Jalalifar MA, Soleimani M, Hajizamani S, Rahim F. Adverse effect of high glucose concentration on stem cell therapy. Int J Hematol Oncol Stem Cell Res. 2013;7(3):34-40.

[40] Jumabay M, Moon JH, Yeerna H, Bostrom KI. Effect of Diabetes Mellitus on Adipocyte-Derived Stem Cells in Rat. J Cell Physiol. 2015;230(11):2821-2828.

[41] Al-Sulaiti H, Dömling AS, Elrayess MA. Mediators of Impaired Adipogenesis in Obesity-Associated Insulin Resistance and T2DM. In: Szablewski L, editor. Adipose Tissue - An Update: IntechOpen; 2019.

[42] Anthonsen MW, Ronnstrand L, Wernstedt C, Degerman E, Holm C. Identification of novel phosphorylation sites in hormone-sensitive lipase that are phosphorylated in response to isoproterenol and govern activation properties in vitro. J Biol Chem. 1998;273(1):215-221.

[43] Hascall V, Wang A. Hyperglycemia diverts dividing stem cells to pathological adipogenesis. Stem Cell Res Ther. 2014;5(6):128.

[44] Han CY, Subramanian S, Chan CK, Omer M, Chiba T, Wight TN, et al. Adipocyte-derived serum amyloid A3 and hyaluronan play a role in monocyte recruitment and adhesion. Diabetes. 2007;56(9):2260-2273.

[45] Makki K, Froguel P, Wolowczuk I. Adipose tissue in

obesity-related inflammation and insulin resistance: cells, cytokines, and chemokines. ISRN Inflamm. 2013;2013:139239.

[46] Liu LF, Craig CM, Tolentino LL, Choi O, Morton J, Rivas H, et al. Adipose tissue macrophages impair preadipocyte differentiation in humans. PLoS One. 2017;12(2):e0170728.

[47] Almuraikhy S, Kafienah W, Bashah M, Diboun I, Jaganjac M, Al-Khelaifi F, et al. Interleukin-6 induces impairment in human subcutaneous adipogenesis in obesity-associated insulin resistance. Diabetologia. 2016;59(11):2406-2416.

[48] Muir LA, Baker NA, Washabaugh AR, Neeley CK, Flesher CG, DelProposto JB, et al. Adipocyte hypertrophy-hyperplasia balance contributes to weight loss after bariatric surgery. Adipocyte. 2017;6(2):134-140.

[49] Mitterberger MC, Mattesich M, Zwerschke W. Bariatric surgery and diet-induced long-term caloric restriction protect subcutaneous adipose-derived stromal/progenitor cells and prolong their life span in formerly obese humans. Exp Gerontol. 2014;56:106-113.

[50] Silva KR, Liechocki S, Carneiro JR, Claudio-da-Silva C, Maya-Monteiro CM, Borojevic R, et al. Stromal-vascular fraction content and adipose stem cell behavior are altered in morbid obese and post bariatric surgery ex-obese women. Stem Cell Res Ther. 2015;6:72.

[51] Vyas KS, Bole M, Vasconez HC, Banuelos JM, Martinez-Jorge J, Tran N, et al. Profile of Adipose-Derived Stem Cells in Obese and Lean Environments. Aesthetic Plast Surg. 2019;43(6):1635-1645.

[52] Timofte D, Mocanu V, Eloae FZ, Hristov I, Cretu IS, Aursulesei V, et al. Immunohistochemical Expression of Growth Hormone Secretagogue Receptor (GSH-R) of Adipose Tissue Macrophagesin Obese Bariatric Patients. Revista de Chimie. 2019;70(9):3428-3430.

[53] Jorgensen NB, Jacobsen SH, Dirksen C, Bojsen-Moller KN, Naver L, Hvolris L, et al. Acute and long-term effects of Roux-en-Y gastric bypass on glucose metabolism in subjects with Type 2 diabetes and normal glucose tolerance. Am J Physiol Endocrinol Metab. 2012;303(1):E122–E131.

[54] Buchwald H, Avidor Y, Braunwald E, Jensen MD, Pories W, Fahrbach K, et al. Bariatric surgery: a systematic review and meta-analysis. JAMA. 2004;292(14):1724-1737.

[55] Schauer PR, Burguera B, Ikramuddin S, Cottam D, Gourash W, Hamad G, et al. Effect of laparoscopic Roux-en Y gastric bypass on type 2 diabetes mellitus. Ann Surg. 2003;238(4):467-484; discussion 84-5.

[56] Cancello R, Henegar C, Viguerie N, Taleb S, Poitou C, Rouault C, et al. Reduction of macrophage infiltration and chemoattractant gene expression changes in white adipose tissue of morbidly obese subjects after surgery-induced weight loss. Diabetes. 2005;54(8):2277-2286.

[57] Labrecque J, Laforest S, Michaud A, Biertho L, Tchernof A. Impact of Bariatric Surgery on White Adipose Tissue Inflammation. Can J Diabetes. 2017;41(4):407-417.

[58] Trachta P, Dostalova I, Haluzikova D, Kasalicky M, Kavalkova P, Drapalova J, et al. Laparoscopic sleeve gastrectomy ameliorates mRNA expression of inflammation-related genes in subcutaneous adipose tissue but not in peripheral monocytes of obese patients. Mol Cell Endocrinol. 2014;383(1-2):96-102.

[59] Haluzikova D, Lacinova Z, Kavalkova P, Drapalova J, Krizova J, Bartlova M, et al. Laparoscopic sleeve gastrectomy differentially affects serum concentrations of FGF-19 and FGF-21 in morbidly obese subjects. Obesity (Silver Spring). 2013;21(7):1335-1342.

[60] Bertola A, Deveaux V, Bonnafous S, Rousseau D, Anty R, Wakkach A, et al. Elevated expression of osteopontin may be related to adipose tissue macrophage accumulation and liver steatosis in morbid obesity. Diabetes. 2009;58(1):125-133.

[61] Burhans MS, Hagman DK, Kuzma JN, Schmidt KA, Kratz M. Contribution of Adipose Tissue Inflammation to the Development of Type 2 Diabetes Mellitus. Compr Physiol. 2018;9(1):1-58.

[62] Liu F, He J, Wang H, Zhu D, Bi Y. Adipose Morphology: a Critical Factor in Regulation of Human Metabolic Diseases and Adipose Tissue Dysfunction. Obes Surg. 2020;30(12):5086-5100.

[63] Tchoukalova YD, Votruba SB, Tchkonia T, Giorgadze N, Kirkland JL, Jensen MD. Regional differences in cellular mechanisms of adipose tissue gain with overfeeding. Proc Natl Acad Sci U S A. 2010;107(42):18226-18231.

[64] Dadson P, Rebelos E, Honka H, Juárez-Orozco LE, Kalliokoski KK, Iozzo P, et al. Change in abdominal, but not femoral subcutaneous fat CT-radiodensity is associated with improved metabolic profile after bariatric surgery. Nutrition, Metabolism and Cardiovascular Diseases. 2020;30(12):2363-2371.

[65] Rosenquist KJ, Pedley A, Massaro JM, Therkelsen KE, Murabito JM, Hoffmann U, et al. Visceral and subcutaneous fat quality and cardiometabolic risk. JACC Cardiovasc Imaging. 2013;6(7):762-771.

Chapter 3

Psychological Considerations for Bariatric Surgery

Anna Guerrini Usubini, Roberto Cattivelli, Valentina Villa, Giorgia Varallo, Valentina Granese, Giada Pietrabissa, Gian Mauro Manzoni, Gianluca Castelnuovo and Enrico Molinari

Abstract

Obesity management requires a multidisciplinary, integrated treatment composed of medical, nutritional, physical, and psychological interventions. Currently, bariatric surgery is the most suitable treatment available in case of severe obesity, or obesity with comorbid medical conditions. Despite bariatric surgery results in a significant weight loss in most of the cases, a not-inconsiderable portion of patients does not achieve relevant outcomes, in terms of limited weight loss or weight regain due to psychological problems. The pre-operative evaluation of the psychological conditions of the candidates for bariatric interventions and pre/post-surgical psychological support is required in order to achieve the desired post-operative outcomes for a long time. In this chapter, we will elucidate the core components of the psychological assessment of bariatric candidates. Moreover, the main directions for the pre/post-surgery psychological support will be provided.

Keywords: obesity, obesity management, bariatric surgery, psychological assessment, psychological support

1. Introduction

Bariatric surgery is the most effective option for individuals with severe obesity. It includes several surgical procedures, commonly divided into restrictive such as Laparoscopic Adjustable Gastric Banding, Banded Gastric Bypass, Sleeve Gastrectomy, malabsorptive such as Biliopancreatic Diversion, Intragastric Balloon, and mixed procedures such as Roux-en-Y- Gastric Bypass, Mini Gastric Bypass, and Gastric Bypass.

Bariatric surgery procedures lead to substantial weight loss and marked improvements in obesity-related comorbidities as well as quality of life. Nonetheless, there is a significant variation in long-term weight loss maintenance and weight regain has been partially attributed to psychological factors.

For these reasons, the pre-operative evaluation of the psychological conditions of the candidates for bariatric interventions is required in order to achieve the desired post-operative outcomes for a long time. In addition, adjunctive pre or post-operative psychosocial interventions are highly recommended for bariatric patients [1, 2] with psychological difficulties.

Within this chapter, the main components of pre-surgical psychological assessment for bariatric candidates will be discussed, including procedures and instruments involved. Moreover, an overview of the principal characteristics of pre/post-surgical psychological support will be provided.

2. Assessment for bariatric candidates

Bariatric surgery has become a popular treatment option for the management of obesity. However, not every obese individual could be considered as a candidate for bariatric surgery. The National Institutes of Health (NIH) Consensus Development Conference Panel held in 1951 outlined criteria for patients considering for bariatric surgery:

- BMI > 40 (obesity grade III); BMI > 35 (obesity grade II) with comorbidities; BMI > 30 (obesity grade I with uncontrolled Diabetes Mellitus type 2 and high cardiovascular risk)

- Reported previous failure of nonsurgical weight-loss efforts

- Absence of medical or psychological contraindications

- Being well-informed, motivated, and compliant

A pre-surgical evaluation of the candidates to bariatric surgery should be conducted in order to assess the presence of recommended criteria for surgery, and to identify and modify, when possible, any risk factors associated with undesired treatment outcomes that may reduce the long term-successful weight loss.

3. Psychological assessment for bariatric surgery candidates

Within the pre-surgical evaluation, the psychological assessment of candidates for bariatric surgery is an essential component. The rationale for the evaluation for bariatric surgery candidates was based on collecting evidences suggesting the presence of a higher level of psychiatric disorders among obese patients than the normative population [3]. The principal goals of psychological pre-surgical evaluation are:

- to identify any psychosocial contraindications to surgery and obstacles to post-operative success, or any psychosocial factor predicting previous weight gain prior to surgery;

- to screen candidates who may benefit from a psychological treatment prior to surgery, in order to maximize long term bariatric outcomes and improve their quality of life;

- to select patients who may need further psychological support after surgery;

- to propose alternative treatment when patients do not meet the criteria for bariatric surgery [4].

4. Psychological conditions of bariatric surgery patients

According to a recent systematic review [5] about one-third of bariatric surgery candidates present a psychological disturbance, such as depression and anxiety and there is a high prevalence of Binge Eating Disorder [6]. Other mental health conditions related to bariatric candidates are psychosis, PTSD substance abuse and personality disorders.

Although the prevalence of mental health conditions among bariatric patients is higher than in the normative population, there is no clear evidence that pre-operative mental health conditions are associated with poorer post-operative weight loss [7]. Nevertheless, prospective studies showed that pre-operative depression and anxiety predict poorer outcomes after surgery [6].

Unfortunately, long term successful weight loss could be less than optimal, and partially depends on the individual's ability to implement consistent lifestyle changes. For these reasons the psychological evaluation of bariatric surgery candidates is requested for monitoring and addressing psychological factors pre-and-post surgery.

In a recent review [8] aimed to explore the present practices adopted by clinics to assess bariatric candidates, it has been highlighted that, in many cases, the presence of uncontrolled symptoms of schizophrenia, drug and alcohol abuse, mental retardation and lack of knowledge about surgery are considered contraindications to surgical approval. Other factors that most frequently are considered limitations to surgery include the presence of symptoms of bipolar disorder and history of suicide attempts, lack of compliance to medical recommendations, unrealistic expectation to surgery outcome, while the age of patients as well as the lack of social support are often considered no-contraindication to surgery. Possible contraindications that could represent a limitation to surgery are past criminal behaviors, the presence of eating disorders, and the inability to follow a diet over time. Finally, according to the programs included in the study, binge eating disorder, depression, obsessive–compulsive disorder, tobacco use, and history of sexual abuse are considered definite or possible contraindication to surgery.

5. The current practices of pre-surgical psychological evaluation

Although the relevance of the psychological assessment for bariatric surgery candidates was recognized for a long time, currently no evidence-based guidelines are available [9, 10].

According to the most commonly used practices in surgery clinics, the evaluation of candidates for bariatric surgery comprises a medical chart review, a comprehensive clinical interview, and psychological testing [11]. Moreover, the psychological assessment should be part of a multidisciplinary approach aimed to carefully assess risks and benefits for the patients related to surgery.

Clinical interviews are commonly used in bariatric centers. During the interview, several areas of interests should be properly investigated:

- Patient's understanding of the surgery

  Patients seeking bariatric surgery are required to have adequate knowledge about the surgery procedures, including which are the potential risks associated with surgery, as well as the lifelong behavioral change that must occur for achieving expected results. For these reasons, during the presurgical psychological evaluation, it is important to know which are the patient's expectation to surgery and assess their willingness to engage themselves in a stable lifestyle behavioral change.

- Eating behaviors

  Among the obese population, there is a high prevalence of individuals with comorbid Binge Eating Disorder (BED), mainly characterized by frequent episodes of binge eating in the absence of following compensatory strategies such as vomiting or purging. Other common eating disorders are Bulimia Nervosa (BN) and Night Eating Syndrome (NES). BM refers to recurrent binge episodes associated with compensatory extreme weight-control behaviors such as vomiting, purging, strict dieting, excessive physical activity. NES consists of morning anorexia, evening hyperphagia, and insomnia. Patients with an eating disorder need to understand that surgery alone cannot modify their problematic eating behaviors, but further efforts in changing their lifestyle behaviors related to eating and physical activity are required in order to achieve lifelong weight loss.

- Psychiatric conditions

  Any previous or current psychiatric disturbance should be addressed during the pre-surgical assessment. The evaluation for psychiatric disorders is aimed to identify symptoms of depression, anxiety, mania, psychosis, suicidal ideation, substance abuse, history of abuse or familial history of mental health problems and previous treatment experienced. Diverse opinions exist about the influence of psychiatric disturbances on surgery outcomes. According to some authors, the presence of one or more mentioned psychiatric disturbances alone is not a contraindication for bariatric surgery. However, it is important to evaluate the severity of symptomatology and, if necessary, referring patients for additional psychological support previous to surgery. Other authors suggest that the presence of uncontrolled eating, current substance abuse, poor adherence to recommendation, psychosis, severe mood disorders, major life stressors should be considered as contraindications to bariatric surgery [12, 13].

- Social support

  Given the impact that surgery will have not only on their lives but also on the environment where patients live, during the psychological assessment clinicians should explore the familial and the social context that surrounds patients. Candidates should be asked to describe the people who live with them, their opinion relative to bariatric surgery decision and whether their family will help them after surgery. Patients should be informed about the possible social consequences that may occur after surgery.

6. Principal interviews and tests available for the assessment of bariatric candidates

There is an availability of templates for conducting interviews that help clinicians to assess the domains of interest.

- The Weight and Lifestyle Inventory [14] is designed to assess the eating and physical activity habits, the psychological status and the presence of stressful life events.

- The Boston Interview [15] aims to assess weight, diet, and nutrition history, dysfunctional eating, medical condition, understanding of surgical procedures, concerns and benefits, motivation for surgery, interpersonal functioning, and psychiatric conditions.

While clinical interviews are widely used in clinical settings, only a few clinics employ some forms of objective tests. The use of psychological instruments allows clinicians to collect more information, in a rapid but precise validated and empirical way than clinical interviews alone. Some broadband instruments provide a broad assessment of patients, across several psychological domains, including emotional, cognitive and behavioral ones. Unfortunately, broadband instruments cannot provide information about specific content areas, such as eating disorders, and require costs for administration. To overcome these limitations, clinicians can administer narrowband instruments that provide a good solution to assess specific domains. In addition, narrowband instruments are more feasible and can be administered quickly. Below is the description of the most frequently used broadband and narrowband instruments for the psychological evaluation of bariatric candidates.

- Minnesota Multiphasic Personality Inventory (MMPI-2; [16]) is the most widely used instruments for the assessment of surgery candidates. It consists of 587 items and it can be administered in two hours approximately, while the newer version, MMPI-2 Restructured Form (MMPI-2 RF; [17]) is composed of 338 items and the time for administration is 35–50 minutes. MMPI-2 RF allows clinicians to assess the global functioning of patients, including thoughts emotions and behaviors. The test allows also to detect cognitive, interpersonal, and somatic problems.

- Symptom Item Checklist–90 –Revised (SCL–90 –R; [18]). The SCL-90 –R is widely used to assess the global psychological distress by exploring nine dimensions: somatization, depression, anxiety, phobic anxiety, obsessive–compulsive, interpersonal sensitivity, hostility, psychoticism, and paranoid ideation. The higher scores reflect higher distress. It is composed of Likert scale-90 items in which symptoms are presented and patients are asked to report how many times they experienced each symptom in the past 7 days.

- Beck Depression Inventory-II (BDI-II; [19]) is a self-report measure composed of 21 items assessing the presence of depressive symptoms.

- Beck Anxiety Inventory (BAI; [20]). is a self-report measure composed of 21 items assessing the presence of anxiety symptoms.

- Binge Eating Scale (BES; [21]). It is one of the most common instruments used among the bariatric population. It is composed of 16 self-report items assessing binge eating severity.

- The Eating Disorders Inventory–III (EDI-III; [22]); It consists of 91 items related to 11 subscales: bulimia, thinness, body dissatisfaction, ineffectiveness, perfectionism, interpersonal distrust, interoceptive awareness, maturity fears, asceticism, impulse regulation, and social insecurity.

Below, a table to describe the most widely used tests is presented in **Table 1**.

	Number of item	Time for administration	Subscales/Key areas
Personality assessment			
MMPI 2	567	90–120 min	Response attitudes, mental health symptoms, personality traits, and special problems 10 clinical scales and 6 validity scales. Domains: personality traits, mental health symptoms, special problems, response attitudes
MMPI-2-RF	338	35–50 min	42 substantive scales and 9 validity scales. Domains: problems, interests, personality psychopathology
SCL-90-R	90	12–15 min	Global psychological distress. 9 Scales: somatization, obsessive–compulsive, interpersonal sensitivity, depression, anxiety, anger/hostility, phobic anxiety, paranoid ideation, psychoticism
PAI	344	50–60 min	11 clinical scales assessing psychopathology in three spectrums: neurotic, psychotic, and behavioral/ impulse control; 5 Treatment scales assessing risk for self-harm or harm to others, how patients respond to environmental factors, and motivation for treatment; 2 interpersonal scales assessing warm/affiliative versus cold/rejecting and dominating/controlling versus submissive; 4 validity scales
MBMD	165	20–25 min	32 clinical scales and 5 validity scales. Domains: response patterns, negative health habits, psychiatric indications, coping styles, and stress moderators
MCMI-III	175	25–30 min	14 personality disorders; 10 clinical syndromes; 5 validity scales
BPI	240	35 min	12 clinical scales: Hypochondriasis, Depression, Denial, Interpersonal Problems, Alienation, Persecutory Ideas, Anxiety, Thinking Disorder, Impulse Expression, Social Introversion, Self-Depreciation, and Deviation; 2 validity scales
Eating disorders			
EDI-3	91	20 min	11 subscales: drive for thinness, bulimia, body dissatisfaction, ineffectiveness, perfectionism, interpersonal distrust, interoceptive awareness, maturity fears, asceticism, impulse regulation, and social insecurity
EDE-Q	32	5–10 min	Eating behaviors. Subscales: restraint, eating concern, weight concern, and shape concern
QEWP	28	5 min	Binge eating patterns
TFEQ	51	20 min	Cognitive and behavioral components of eating. 3 scales: restraint, hunger, and disinhibition
BES	16	5 min	Symptoms of Binge Eating
NEQ	14	5–10 min	Symptoms of night eating syndrome. 4 scales: nocturnal ingestion, evening hyperphagia, morning anorexic, and mood/sleep
Mood Disturbances			
BDI-II	21	5–10 min	Symptomps of depression
BAI	21	5–10 min	Symptoms of anxiety
PHQ-9	9	5 min	Symptoms of depression

	Number of item	Time for administration	Subscales/Key areas
CES-D	20	10 min	Symptoms of depression
MDQ	13	5 min	Bipolar symptoms
GAD-7	7	5 min	Symptoms of anxiety
Substance abuse			
AUDIT	10	5 min	Drinking patterns
MAST	25	5–10 min	Alchool abuse and related problems
SASSI-3	93	20 min	Substance abuse. 8 subscales: symptoms of substance misuse, obvious attributes, subtle attributes, defensiveness, supplemental addiction measure, family versus control subjects, correctional, and random answering pattern
Quality of life			
IWQL	74	15 min	8 domains: health, social/interpersonal life, work, mobility, self-esteem, sexual life, activities of daily living, comfort with food
Cognitive development			
MMSE	30	10 min	Cognitive impairment. Domains: orientation, attention, registration, recall, language, repetition, complex commands.
Physical conditions			
MBHI	150	20 min	Personality and Coping style among people with physical pathologies. 8 coping style scales; six psychogenic attitudes; 3 psychosomatic correlate scales; 3 risk for poorer outcomes scales.

Abbreviations: MMPI-2; Minnesota Multiphasic Personality Inventory 2; MMPI-2-RF: Minnesota Multiphasic Personality Inventory-2-Revised Form; SCL-90-R. Symptom Check-List-90-Revised; PAI: Personality Assessment Inventory; MBMD: Millon Behavioral Medicine Diagnostic; MCMI-III: Millon Clinical Multiaxial Inventory; BPI: Basic Personality Inventory; EDI-3: Eating Disorders Inventory; EDE-Q: Eating Disorder Examination-Questionnaire; QEWP: Questionnaire of Eating and Weight Patterns–Revised; TFEQ: The Three-Factor Eating Questionnaire; BES: Binge Eating Scale; NEQ: Night eating Questionnaire; BDI-III: Beck Depression inventory; BAI: Beck Anxiety Inventory; PHQ-9: The Patient Health Questionnaire-9; CES-D: Center for Epidemiologic Studies Depression Scale; MDQ: Mood Disorders Questionnaire; GAD-7: Generalized Anxiety Disorder-7; AUDIT: Alcohol Use Disorders Identification Test; MAST: Michigan Alcoholism Screening Test; SASSI-3: Substance Abuse Subtle Screening Inventory-3; IWQOL: Impact of Weight on Quality of Life; MMSE: Mini-Mental State Evaluation; MBHI: Millon Behavioral Health Inventory.

Table 1.
Principal used psychometric instruments for the assessment of bariatric candidates.

7. Psychological pre/post-surgical intervention for bariatric candidates

Bariatric surgery is the most effective intervention for weight loss in the field of obesity management. Unfortunately, patients often do not achieve optimal results in term of weight loss maintenance over time and meet various difficulties related to eating behaviors and psychological functioning. Given the significant variation in weight long-term outcomes after surgery that could be partially attributed to a number of risk factors, including psychological factors, psychological pre-operative or post-operative interventions are increasingly being recommended for patients seeking or undergoing bariatric surgery [23].

The most delivered psychological interventions included Cognitive Behavioral Therapy (CBT) but promising evidence suggests the effectiveness of intervention based on Acceptance and Commitment Therapy (ACT) and Dialectical Behavioral Therapy (DBT).

Cognitive behavioral interventions typically include psychoeducation, goal setting, self-monitoring, stimulus control, problem solving, and reinforcement, for the promotion of lifestyle-related behavior change. Through the psychological intervention, patients are encouraged to recognize their problematic eating behaviors, learn strategies to cope with life stressors, and engage themselves in healthy eating behaviors and physical activity. Recently, David and colleagues [5] conducted a systematic review aimed to examine the effectiveness of cognitive behavioral interventions. Results showed that the most common techniques employed during the interventions were psychoeducation, self-monitoring, goal setting, stimulus control, cognitive restructuring, problem solving and reinforcement, as well as addressing ambivalence, improving self-care and prevention of relapse. Most of the interventions included in the study were delivered in person, or in combination with telephone or web. With respect to intervention outcomes, the main findings of the review revealed that 32% of included studies showed a significant impact on weight loss. Specifically, it seems that the higher impact on weight loss was found in post-operative intervention, than the benefits of pre-operative interventions which were not maintained at follow-up. Other interventions outcomes were lifestyle behaviors, eating pathology, and psychological functioning. Results showed that psychological interventions seem to have an inconsistent influence on change in dietary habits and physical activity, but a limited number of studies examined this outcome. With respect to eating pathology, psychological interventions included in the study revealed a significant impact on reducing binge eating and emotional eating. Similarly, interventions had a positive impact on psychological functioning. Both pre-operative and post-operative interventions improved quality of life and reduced depression and anxiety symptoms.

Recently, other forms of psychological interventions were applied to bariatric patients. In a pilot RCT, Weineland and colleagues [24] compared an intervention based on ACT (two face to face session in combination with internet-based support) to usual treatment. Results showed that patients in the ACT condition significantly improved in eating disorders, body dissatisfaction, quality of life, and acceptance of thoughts and feelings related to weight.

Promising results were also obtained in an observational study [25] in which a pre-operative intervention based on DBT skills training combined with treatment as usual compared to a treatment as usual group. The intervention of DBT was focused on regulating emotions with emotion regulation, mindfulness, distress tolerance, and interpersonal effectiveness training. The results offered preliminary evidence in support of the effectiveness of a brief DBT skills training intervention in combination with treatment as usual in reducing eating pathology (binge eating and emotional eating).

8. Conclusions

Bariatric surgery has been demonstrated to be a valid solution for the treatment of obesity. It is recommended for well-motivated and informed patients with severe obesity or obesity with related comorbidities. Approximately, all bariatric surgery procedures are effective in producing weight loss and related substantial improvements in health conditions [26–28].

Candidates for bariatric surgery require not only a multidisciplinary pre-operative screening, which is aimed to prepare and educate patients for the lifestyle changes required after surgery, but also would benefit from a supportive, integrated additional psychological interventions aimed to maximize weight loss and weight loss maintenance after surgery. Particularly, weight loss is not the primary goal of psychological interventions. In fact, findings indicate that the pre-operative interventions do not have a significant effect on weight loss [29]. Rather, they should be considered an option for patients to overcome their difficulties, reduce pre-existing symptomatology, and improving in their eating behaviors and lifestyle. On the contrary, psychological post-operative interventions have been associated with significant weight loss and currently they are the most promising approach to improve the outcomes of bariatric surgery.

Author details

Anna Guerrini Usubini[1,2], Roberto Cattivelli[1,2]*, Valentina Villa[1], Giorgia Varallo[1,2], Valentina Granese[1,2], Giada Pietrabissa[1,2], Gian Mauro Manzoni[1,3], Gianluca Castelnuovo[1,2] and Enrico Molinari[1,2]

1 Istituto Auxologico Italiano IRCCS, Psychology Research Laboratory, Italy

2 Department of Psychology, Catholic University of Milan, Italy

3 Faculty of Psychology, eCampus University, Italy

*Address all correspondence to: r.cattivelli@auxologico.it

References

[1] Kalarchian MA, Marcus MD. Psychosocial concerns following bariatric surgery: Current status. Current Obesity Reports. 2019;*8*(1):1-9 https://doi.org/10.1007/s13679-019-0325-3

[2] Velapati, S. R., Shah, M., Kuchkuntla, A. R., Abu-dayyeh, B., Grothe, K., Hurt, R. T., & Mundi, M. S. (2018). Weight Regain After Bariatric Surgery: Prevalence, Etiology, and Treatment. In *Current Nutrition Reports* (Vol. 7, Issue 4, pp. 329-334). Current Science Inc. https://doi.org/10.1007/s13668-018-0243-0

[3] Dixon JB, Dixon ME, O'Brien PE. Depression in association with severe obesity: Changes with weight loss. Archives of Internal Medicine. 2003;*163*(17):2058-2065 https://doi.org/10.1001/archinte.163.17.2058

[4] Block AR, Sarwer DB. Presurgical psychological screening: Understanding patients, improving outcomes. In: Block AR, Sarwer DB, editors. *Presurgical Psychological Screening: Understanding Patients, Improving Outcomes*. American Psychological Association; 2013 https://doi.org/10.1037/14035-000

[5] David LA, Sijercic I, Cassin SE. Preoperative and post-operative psychosocial interventions for bariatric surgery patients: A systematic review. Obesity Reviews. 2020 https://doi.org/10.1111/obr.12926

[6] Kalarchian MA, King WC, Devlin MJ, Hinerman A, Marcus MD, Yanovski SZ, et al. Mental disorders and weight change in a prospective study of bariatric surgery patients: 7 years of follow-up. Surgery for Obesity and Related Diseases. 2019 https://doi.org/10.1016/j.soard.2019.01.008

[7] Dawes AJ, Maggard-Gibbons M, Maher AR, Booth MJ, Miake-Lye I, Beroes JM, et al. Mental health conditions among patients seeking and undergoing bariatric surgery a meta-analysis. JAMA - Journal of the American Medical Association. 2016. DOI: 10.1001/jama.2015.18118

[8] Bauchowitz, A. U., Gonder-Frederick, L. A., Olbrisch, M. E., Azarbad, L., Ryee, M. Y., Woodson, M., Miller, A., & Schirmer, B. (2005). Psychosocial evaluation of bariatric surgery candidates: A survey of present practices. In *Psychosomatic Medicine* (Vol. 67, Issue 5, pp. 825-832). Psychosom Med. https://doi.org/10.1097/01.psy.0000174173.32271.01

[9] Fabricatore AN, Crerand CE, Wadden TA, Sarwer DB, Krasucki JL. How do mental health professionals evaluate candidates for bariatric surgery? Survey results. Obesity Surgery. 2006;**16**(5):567-573 https://doi.org/10.1381/096089206776944986

[10] Flores, C. A. it. (2014). Psychological assessment for bariatric surgery: current practices. In *Arquivos brasileiros de cirurgia digestiva : ABCD = Brazilian archives of digestive surgery* (Vol. 27, Issue Suppl 1, pp. 59-62). Colégio Brasileiro de Cirurgia Digestiva. https://doi.org/10.1590/s0102-6720201400s100015

[11] Marek RJ, Heinberg LJ, Lavery M, Merrell Rish J, Ashton K. A review of psychological assessment instruments for use in bariatric surgery evaluations. Psychological Assessment. 2016;*28*(9):1142-1157 https://doi.org/10.1037/pas0000286

[12] Edwards-Hampton, S. A., & Wedin, S. (2015). Preoperative psychological assessment of patients seeking weight-loss surgery: Identifying challenges and solutions. In *Psychology Research and Behavior Management* (Vol. 8, pp.

263-272). Dove Medical Press Ltd. https://doi.org/10.2147/PRBM.S69132

[13] Marihart CL, Brunt AR, Geraci AA. Older adults fighting obesity with bariatric surgery: Benefits, side effects, and outcomes. SAGE Open Medicine. 2014;*2*:205031211453091 https://doi.org/10.1177/2050312114530917

[14] Wadden, T. A., & Foster, G. D. (2006). Weight and Lifestyle Inventory (WALI). In *Obesity (Silver Spring, Md.): Vol. 14 Suppl 2*. Obesity (Silver Spring). https://doi.org/10.1038/oby.2006.289

[15] Sogg S, Mori DL. Revising the Boston interview: Incorporating new knowledge and experience. Surgery for Obesity and Related Diseases. 2008;*4*(3):455-463.e20 https://doi.org/10.1016/j.soard.2008.01.007

[16] Butcher JN. Minnesota Multiphasic Personality Inventory. In *The Corsini Encyclopedia of Psychology* (pp. 1-3). Inc: John Wiley & Sons; 2010 https://doi.org/10.1002/9780470479216.corpsy0573

[17] Marek RJ, Block AR, Ben-Porath YS. The Minnesota multiphasic personality inventory-2-restructured form (MMPI-2-RF): Incremental validity in predicting early postoperative outcomes in spine surgery candidates. Psychological Assessment. 2015;*27*(1):114-124 https://doi.org/10.1037/pas0000035

[18] Derogatis LR, Unger R. Symptom Checklist-90-Revised. In *The Corsini Encyclopedia of Psychology* (pp. 1-2). Inc: John Wiley & Sons; 2010 https://doi.org/10.1002/9780470479216.corpsy0970

[19] Beck, A. T., Steer, R. A., & Brown, G. (1996). Beck depression inventory–II. Psychological Assessment. ?

[20] Steer, R. A., & Beck, A. T. (1997). Beck Anxiety Inventory. ?

[21] Gormally J, Black S, Daston S, Rardin D. The assessment of binge eating severity among obese persons. Addictive Behaviors. 1982;*7*(1):47-55 https://doi.org/10.1016/0306-4603(82)90024-7

[22] Garner, D. M. (n.d.). *Eating Disorder Inventory ™-3 (EDI ™-3)*.

[23] Mitchell JE, Christian NJ, Flum DR, Pomp A, Pories WJ, Wolfe BM, et al. Postoperative behavioral variables and weight change 3 years after bariatric surgery. JAMA Surgery. 2016;*151*(8):752-757 https://doi.org/10.1001/jamasurg.2016.0395

[24] Weineland S, Arvidsson D, Kakoulidis TP, Dahl J. Acceptance and commitment therapy for bariatric surgery patients, a pilot RCT. Obesity Research and Clinical Practice. 2012;*6*(1) https://doi.org/10.1016/j.orcp.2011.04.004

[25] Delparte CA, Power HA, Gelinas BL, Oliver AM, Hart RD, Wright KD. Examination of the Effectiveness of a Brief, Adapted Dialectical Behavior Therapy-Skills Training Group for Bariatric Surgical Candidates. *Springer*; 2018 https://doi.org/10.1007/s11695-018-3515-2

[26] Biter LU, van Buuren MMA, Mannaerts GHH, Apers JA, Dunkelgrün M, Vijgen GHEJ. Quality of life 1 year after laparoscopic sleeve Gastrectomy versus laparoscopic roux-en-Y gastric bypass: A randomized controlled trial focusing on Gastroesophageal reflux disease. Obesity Surgery. 2017;*27*(10):2557-2565 https://doi.org/10.1007/s11695-017-2688-4

[27] Flølo TN, Andersen JR, Kolotkin RL, Aasprang A, Natvig GK, Hufthammer KO, et al. Five-year outcomes after vertical sleeve Gastrectomy for severe obesity: A prospective cohort study. Obesity Surgery. 2017;*27*(8):1944-1951 https://doi.org/10.1007/s11695-017-2605-x

[28] Porta A, Aiolfi A, Musolino C, Antonini I, Zappa MA. Prospective comparison and quality of life for single-incision and conventional laparoscopic sleeve Gastrectomy in a series of morbidly obese patients. Obesity Surgery. 2017;*27*(3):681-687 https://doi.org/10.1007/s11695-016-2338-2

[29] Rudolph A, Hilbert A. Post-operative behavioural management in bariatric surgery: A systematic review and meta-analysis of randomized controlled trials. Obesity Reviews. 2013;*14*(4):292-302 https://doi.org/10.1111/obr.12013

Chapter 4

Nutritional Deficiencies Post Bariatric Surgery: A Forgotten Area Impacting Long-Term Success and Quality of Life

Wahiba Elhag and Walid El Ansari

Abstract

Bariatric surgery (BS) results in significant weight loss and improvement of obesity associated comorbidities. Despite the benefits achieved with these operations, deficiencies of vitamins and other micronutrients are common. Such deficiencies may become clinically significant if not discovered and treated early. Therefore, it is imperative to undertake thorough screening, and have sound preventive strategies in place in order to make BS a safer procedure. This chapter will provide the multidisciplinary bariatric team with a comprehensive review of micronutrient deficiencies before and after bariatric surgery. The focus will be on the most common micronutrient deficiencies that are encountered in various types of BS procedures, including water soluble vitamins, fat-soluble vitamins, minerals and trace elements deficiencies, as well as protein malnutrition. The chapter starts with an overview of the causes of micronutrient deficiencies in patients with obesity and before undergoing BS. It reviews the screening of patients for preexisting micronutrient deficiencies prior to their BS. Then the chapter addresses the potential causes and mechanisms leading to such deficiencies after BS. It then conducts an in depth discourse of the prevalence of deficiencies by the type of BS, the presenting symptoms, and the investigations required for the diagnoses. The chapter will also discuss the management of each deficiency according to the severity of the symptoms. The chapter also reviews the recent updated guidelines for standard nutritional care post BS. We will finally conclude with a framework of the preventive strategies for optimal care to ensure long term success post-surgery.

Keywords: obesity, bariatric surgery, micronutrients, deficiencies, water soluble vitamins, fat soluble vitamins, minerals, trace elements, protein malnutrition

1. Introduction

Bariatric surgery (BS) has proven to be an effective treatment for weight loss, reducing obesity associated comorbidities, improving quality of life, and reducing mortality rates [1, 2]. The increasing amount of evidence on the benefits of BS has contributed to its increased popularity over the last decade [1]. Despite the proven benefits of BS, it also carries the risk of short- and long-term complications.

IntechOpen

An important complication is the nutritional and micronutrient deficiencies. Nutritional deficiencies can present with a wide range of clinical manifestations, depending on the specific nutrients/micronutrients that are involved, the severity, and the duration of the deficiency states. Additionally, these deficiencies can worsen over time, leading to severe consequences, such as anemia (iron, folate, B12), peripheral neuropathy (folate, B6, B12, copper), Wernicke encephalopathy (B1) and metabolic bone disease (vitamin D, calcium). Therefore, lifelong screening of individuals who had undergone bariatric surgery is critical to identify these complications and treat them effectively to ensure long-term success. This chapter will provide a comprehensive review of these nutritional complications. The chapter will also furnish information about the recommended micronutrient supplementations and nutritional follow-up.

2. Micronutrient deficiencies prior to bariatric surgery

Nutritional deficiencies often exist prior to BS [3–5]. Subjects with obesity typically adopt an unhealthy high calorie, low quality diet with unbalanced nutritional composition [6]. For instance, one study showed that in female BS candidates, despite consumption of high-caloric diet (2801 ± 970 kcal/day), 66% of them had at least a single micronutrient deficiency [7]. Prior to BS, low iron, ferritin, vitamin B12 and hemoglobin were observed among 12.6%, 8.7%, 10.6% and 7.7%, of patients respectively [7]; and the incidence of folate deficiency before BS was 26.8% [8]. Vitamin D deficiency is the most common deficiency in patients undergoing BS with a prevalence as high as 78.8% [7, 8].

Research found that low preoperative levels of hemoglobin, vitamin B12, and ferritin were independently associated with reduction in the levels of micronutrients postoperatively [8]. Moreover, vitamins D and B1 and albumin deficiencies before BS predicted deficiencies one year after surgery [8].

Such findings highlight the need for complete nutritional assessments and adequate correction of pre-existing deficits before BS. Therefore, all BS candidates must undergo appropriate nutritional evaluation, including micronutrient measurements at least once preoperatively. Screening should include iron studies, and vitamins D and B12 and folic acid levels. The repetition of the tests until surgery should be individualized as clinically indicated [9, 10]. In comparison with purely restrictive procedures, more extensive nutritional evaluations are required for malabsorptive procedures. For instance, thiamine and vitamins A and E levels may be assessed in patients prior to Roux en Y gastric bypass (RYGB) and biliopancreatic diversion with duodenal switch (BPD/DS) [10].

Deficiencies found on screening prior to BS should be treated accordingly to avoid worsening of the symptoms post-surgery [9]. For vitamin D, there is a lack of solid evidence regarding the cutoff value where treatment should be started. A group of experts advocated supplementation in all patients with values below 20 ng/mL, and in an individualized manner for values between 21 and 30 ng/mL [9].

3. Micronutrient deficiencies post bariatric surgery

3.1 Causes of micronutrient deficiencies post bariatric surgery

Several factors and mechanisms contribute to the development of nutritional deficiencies post BS. Below are some examples:

3.1.1 Non-compliance with nutritional supplementation

Nonadherence to the recommended nutritional supplementation is recognized as a critical factor that leads to nutritional deficiency after BS. Compliance with multivitamins tends to be good in the early post-surgery period and decreases on the long term. For instance, a study of 16,620 patients post BS showed that the pharmacy dispensing of micronutrient supplements by patients significantly decreased between the first and fifth years for iron (from 27.7 to 24.5%), calcium (from 14·4 to 7·7%), but increased for vitamin D (from 33·1 to 34·7%) [11]. Barriers to vitamin adherence post BS include forgetting to take the supplementation and difficulty in swallowing the pills [12].

3.1.2 Lack of follow up

Despite clear international guidelines, long-term follow-up after BS is poor. A study assessed the follow up with the bariatric surgeon after RYGB and demonstrated a significant increase in the time between follow ups (13.3 ± 7.8 vs. 86.9 ± 39.9 months) in the long-term [13]. The same study demonstrated that a shorter time since last surgeon visit was independently predictive of multivitamin use ($p = 0.001$) [13]. Research also reported that male sex, younger age, absence of type 2 diabetes and poor 1-year follow-up were predictors of poor 5-year follow-up [11].

3.1.3 Other causes

Other contributing factors include pre-operative deficiencies, post-surgery food intolerance, poor eating habits, vomiting, changes in taste and eating patterns [14].

3.2 Mechanisms of micronutrient deficiency after bariatric surgery

The underling mechanisms that contribute to micronutrient deficiency following BS include reduced food intake due to restrictive effect of surgery, rerouting of nutrient flow which affect absorption, and changes in gastrointestinal anatomy/physiology post-surgery. It is important to note that the anatomical changes and the mechanisms of action of the various procedures dictate the frequency and severity of nutritional deficiencies after BS. For instance, micronutrient deficiencies are less common in restrictive procedures such as gastric banding (LAGB) and laparoscopic sleeve gastrectomy (LSG), where there are no alterations of the intestinal continuity and normal digestive processes. However, micronutrient deficiencies are more common after surgical procedures that cause malabsorption such as RYGB, one-anastomosis gastric bypass (OAGB), single anastomosis duodeno–ileal bypass with sleeve gastrectomy (SADI-S) and BPD/DS [10, 15].

3.3 Water soluble vitamin deficiency post bariatric surgery

3.3.1 Vitamin B1 (thiamin)

Vitamin B1 is absorbed in the jejunum and therefore may be excluded from absorption after RYGB and BPD/DS [16]. Additionally, the storage of thiamine is low in the human body and can become rapidly devoid without regular and adequate intake [8]. These characteristics might explain why thiamin deficiency is observed subsequent to a short period of persistent vomiting after surgical complications such as band slippage post LAGB [17], stomach oedema after LSG [18],

Mico/micro deficiency	Clinical features and complications	Management
Vitamin B1 Thiamin	Wernicke encephalopathy (confabulations, ophthalmoplegia, ataxia) Korsakoff syndrome Dry Beriberi (polyneuropathy, paresthesia) Wet Beriberi (cardiomegaly, tachycardia, CHF)	Oral: 100 mg 2–3 times daily until symptoms resolve IV: 200–500 mg once or twice daily for 3–5 d, followed by 250 mg/d for 3–5 d or until symptoms resolve, then 100 mg/d orally, indefinitely, or until risk factors resolve IM: 250 mg once daily for 3–5 d or 100–250 mg monthly
Vitamin B12 Cobalamin	Macrocytic anemia, peripheral and central neuropathy, myelopathy, memory disturbance, dementia, depression, delusions	1000 µg/d to achieve normal levels and then resume dosages recommended to maintain normal levels
Folate	Macrocytic anemia, leukopenia peripheral neuropathy, myelopathy, glossitis, fetal neural defects. May aggravate B12 deficiency	Oral dose of 1 mg of folate daily to reach normal levels and then resume recommended dosage to maintain normal levels
Vitamin A	Ocular xerosis, night blindness, decreased immunity, scaling skin	Vitamin A deficiency without corneal changes: 10,000–25,000 IU/d of vitamin orally until clinical improvement Vitamin A deficiency with corneal changes: 50,000–100,000 IU of vitamin A IM for 3 d, followed by 50,000 IU/d IM for 2 weeks
Vitamin D	Osteomalacia, bone demineralization, increased risk of fractures	Vitamin D3 at least 3000 IU/d and as high as 6000 IU/d, or 50,000 IU vitamin D2 1–3 times weekly
Vitamin E	Hemolytic anemia, peripheral neuropathy, loss of deep tendon reflexes, ataxia, diminished perception of vibration and position ophthalmoplegia, myopathy, rash	Optimal therapeutic dose of Vitamin E for bariatric patients is not defined Potential antioxidant benefits can be achieved with supplements of 100–400 IU/d Additional dose may be required for replacement
Vitamin K	Coagulopathy, excessive bleeding or bruising	Parenteral dose (10 mg) for symptomatic patient acute malabsorption A dose of either 1–2 mg/d orally or 1–2 mg/week parenterally recommended for patients with chronic malabsorption
Iron	Microcytic anemia, fatigue glossitis, nail dystrophy	Oral: 150–200 mg of elemental iron daily to amounts as high as 300 mg 2–3 times daily (ferrous sulfate, fumarate, gluconate) Vitamin C supplementation may be added to increase iron absorption IV iron infusion (ferric gluconate or sucrose forms) for patients with severe intolerance to oral iron or refractory deficiency Blood transfusion for severe iron deficiency anemia
Calcium	Fatigue, arrhythmia, myopathy, bone demineralization	Repletion of calcium deficiency varies by surgical procedure BPD/DS: 1800–2400 mg/d; LAGB, LSG, RYGB: 1200–1500 mg/d
Zinc	Hair loss, pica, dermatitis, chronic diarrhea, dysgeusia, hypogonadism or erectile dysfunction (in males)	Optimal therapeutic dose is unknown. Treatment should target normal biochemical levels. For every 8–15 mg/day elemental zinc provided, 1 mg/day copper should be supplemented to avoid inducing a copper deficiency

Mico/micro deficiency	Clinical features and complications	Management
Copper	Anemia, neutropenia, myeloneuropathy sensory ataxia, impaired wound healing	Treatment varies with severity of deficiency Mild–moderate: 3–8 mg/d oral copper gluconate or sulfate until indices return to normal Severe: 2–4 mg/d intravenous copper can be initiated for 6 d or until serum levels return to normal and neurologic symptoms resolve Copper gluconate or sulfate is recommended
Selenium	Anemia, persistent diarrhea, cardiomyopathy, metabolic bone disease	Optimal therapeutic dose of selenium for bariatric patients is not defined RDA for selenium is 55 micrograms per day

IV intravenous; IM intramuscular; D: day, CHF: congestive heart failure, LAGB laparoscopic gastric band, LSG laparoscopic sleeve gastrectomy, RYGB Roux en Y gastric bypass, BPD/D biliopancreatic diversion.

Table 1.
Summary of common micro and micro nutritional deficiencies.

or stoma stenosis after RYGB [19]. Cases of thiamine deficiencies have also been reported after BPD/DS [20].

The manifestations of thiamine deficiency include peripheral neuropathy, Wernicke's encephalopathy (WE), Korsakoff's psychoses and cardiomyopathy [14, 10] (**Table 1**). These clinical conditions could be severe or even fatal if they are not recognized and treated promptly. Borderline deficiency may cause less severe symptoms that could be missed. Therefore, oral or parenteral thiamine supplementation should be initiated in any bariatric patient presenting with persistent vomiting severe enough to interfere with adequate nutrition, even before obtaining confirmatory laboratory data [10, 14]. In symptomatic patients, oral supplementation may be used only after 1–2 weeks of parenteral administration and continued until symptom resolution [10].

In severely malnourished patients receiving nutrition support, empiric thiamine supplementation along with fluid and electrolyte monitoring and replacement are indicated to avoid exacerbation of thiamin deficiency and refeeding syndrome [10]. Refeeding syndrome is a condition that results from fluid and electrolyte imbalances, particularly hypophosphatemia, causing serious complications such as cardiac arrhythmias [21]. Empiric thiamine supplementation is also indicated for high-risk bariatric patients and patients with risk factors for thiamine deficiency such as females, African Americans, patients not attending the dietitian clinic, patients with gastrointestinal symptoms, heart failure, persistent vomiting, or on parenteral nutrition and those with excessive alcohol use [10]. The recommended dose for prevention and treatment of thiamin deficiency is summarized in **Table 1**.

Wernicke Encephalopathy: is a serious complication of thiamin deficiency. It is an acute neuropsychiatric syndrome characterized by ataxia, ophthalmoparesis, nystagmus, and confusion. WE most commonly occurs during the first weeks to months following BS [17]. Among patients who were diagnosed with WE, 52% had RYGB and 21% had LSG [15]. Symptoms of WE are typically preceded by malnutrition, which results from persistent prolonged vomiting, although vitamin noncompliance or increased alcoholism are also risk factors [15]. Radiologic imaging of the brain especially magnetic resonance imaging can be used to support the diagnosis of WE, but is not always sensitive to WE symptoms. Findings include hyperintensities in the thalamic region, the mammillary bodies, and the region around the third and fourth ventricle [22]. The recommended treatment is 500 mg of parenteral thiamine three times daily until symptoms of acute WE resolute [10]. The treatment is lifesaving and has the potential to reverse this acute neuropsychiatric syndrome. Recovery typically occurs within 3–6 months of initiation of therapy if the symptoms are recognized early [23]. Studies have shown that patients who received suboptimal thiamin dose or had more than one acute symptom were more likely to progress later into a permanent neurologic deficits (Korsakoff's syndrome) [17]. Korsakoff's syndrome is neuropsychiatric disorder characterized by severe amnesia, executive problems, and confabulations, leading to lifelong impairment [17].

3.3.2 Vitamin B12 (cobalamin)

Vitamin B12 (cobalamin) binds to the intrinsic factor, a protein secreted by the stomach. The complex formed is then absorbed by the small intestine [16]. Vitamin B12 deficiency post BS can result from inadequate secretion of intrinsic factor, limited gastric acidity, and most importantly from the bypassing of the duodenum, which is the main site of vitamin B12 absorption [6, 24]. Cobalamin stores in the liver are usually high and therefore vitamin B12 deficiency is rare in the first year after BS; however the incidence tends to increase on the long term [25]. The prevalence vitamin B12 deficiency is 14.3% after LSG and 16% post RYGB [26]. In addition to anemia, vitamin B12 deficiency can cause neurological and psychiatric symptoms [6] (**Table 1**). Therefore, regular screening is required (e.g., every 3 months) in the first year after BS and at least annually after that or as clinically indicated. This is particularly important with chronic use of medications that worsen B12 deficiency such as metformin, proton-pump inhibitors, and seizure medications [10]. In some instances, serum B12 may not be adequate to identify B12 deficiency; in such cases measuring serum methylmalonic acid, with or without homocysteine, should be considered to identify metabolic deficiency of B12, especially in symptomatic or in patients with history of B12 deficiency [10]. Intramuscular or intranasal regimens is preferred over oral supplementation as only 1% of oral vitamin B12 is passively absorbed without intrinsic factor [14].

3.3.3 Folic acid

Complex dietary folates are absorbed throughout the small intestine but mainly at the brush border of the duodenum and upper jejunum [16]. Since folate is absorbed throughout the small intestine, the deficiency is primarily induced by the decrease in dietary intake and to a lesser extent due to malabsorption specially after procedures that bypass the first part small intestine (RYGB, BPD/DS) [6]. Furthermore, folate deficiency can be aggravated by vitamin B12 deficiency since the latter is necessary for the conversion of inactive methyltetrahydrofolic acid to the active tetrahydrofolic acid [6]. The reported prevalence of folate deficiency after LSG and RYGB is 3.6% and 4.2% respectively [26]. Folate deficiency has been associated with a variety of symptoms (**Table 1**) [6, 23]. Maternal folate deficiency in pregnancy can cause fetal neurological abnormalities such as growth retardation, and congenital defects (neural tube) [16, 27]. Therefore, adequate folate supplementation is particularly important after malabsorptive procedures and in women of the childbearing age [10].

3.4 Fat soluble vitamin deficiency post bariatric surgery

3.4.1 Vitamin A

The absorption of vitamin A is reduced after bariatric procedures. The incidence of vitamin A deficiency is 11.1% at one year post LSG [26]. A higher prevalence is reported after malabsorptive procedures where deficiency was found in up to 70% of patients 4 years after RYGB and BPD/DS [28]. This is due to fat malabsorption and steatorrhoea. Therefore, routine fat-soluble vitamin supplementation is recommended in all patients post BPD/DS [10]. The clinical manifestations of vitamin A deficits are night blindness, xerophthalmia and dry hair [6].

3.4.2 Vitamin D

Vitamin D is a fat-soluble vitamin absorbed preferentially in the jejunum and ileum. Hence, a high incidence of vitamin D deficiency in seen after malabsorptive procedures despite routine supplementation [16]. The reported deficiency after LSG and RYGB is 66.7% and 65.4% respectively [26]. The prevalence of post BPD/DS vitamin D deficiency ranged from 37.1% at one year to 50.8% at 6 years [29]. The most important consequence of vitamin D deficiency is bone demineralization. Therefore, despite the absence of conclusive evidence regarding the long-term risk of fractures after BS, calcium and vitamin D routine supplementation is strongly recommended, especially after RYGB and malabsorptive procedures [10, 30]. The standard supplementation is frequently insufficient to maintain adequate vitamin D levels in patients with malabsorption, and much higher oral or parenteral doses may be required [8, 28]. For treatment, vitamin D3 is recommended as it is a more potent than vitamin D2; however, both can be utilized [10].

3.4.3 Vitamin K

Low levels of vitamin K have been observed in 1.8% post RYGB and 7.4% post SADI patients one year after surgery [31]. However, clinical symptoms such as easy bruising, and increased bleeding are rare [6]. Some cases of fetal and newborn intracranial hemorrhage related to maternal vitamin K deficiency have been described after BPD/DS [27], and have been also reported after LAGB in a pregnant woman with prolonged vomiting due to slippage of the gastric band resulting in gastric outlet obstruction [32].

3.4.4 Vitamin E

Vitamin E deficiency after BS is rare. The reported incidence is 4.8% and 0.9% after RYGB and SADI respectively [31, 33]. The most common symptoms associated with vitamin E deficiency include neuropathy, myopathy and anemia [21] (**Table 1**). Vitamin E neuropathy and myopathy can be treated with a dose of vitamin E 400 IU daily.

3.5 Minerals

3.5.1 Iron

Iron deficiency with or without anemia is frequently observed after BS [10]. The incidence after LAGB and LSG ranges between 14 to 18% [10]. The prevalence after RYGB and BPB/DS is 51.3% and 15% respectively [34, 35]. Several mechanisms lead to iron deficiency post BS. First, iron malabsorption can occur as a result of the bypassing of the duodenum and proximal jejunum post BS where most of iron absorption occurs. Second, decreased gastric acidity and accelerated gastric emptying impair the reduction of iron from the ferric (Fe 3+) to the absorbable ferrous state (Fe 2+). Third is the decreased intake of iron-rich foods (meats, vegetables) post BS. Finally, the absorption of iron may be affected by the interaction with other nutritional supplements (e.g., calcium) [10, 14]. Menstruating women are at higher risk for iron deficiency and anemia, specially patients with polymenorrhagia [25]. Other risk factors for iron deficiency include malabsorptive procedures, young age, preoperative anemia and low baseline ferritin level [36]. The clinical features of iron deficiency are summarized in **Table 1**. The measurement of serum ferritin is the best diagnostic test for detecting iron deficiency and a better indicator of iron body capacity as it becomes abnormal prior to the decrease in serum iron concentration [6]. Prophylactic iron supplementation is recommended after all types of BS to minimize the risk of deficiency [10]. Iron is usually included in oral multivitamin and mineral preparations with the inclusion of vitamin C, which will increase iron absorption [10]. They should not be taken along together with calcium supplements as such supplements may affect the absorption of iron. Severe cases of iron deficiency anemia require intravenous iron or blood transfusion [36].

3.5.2 Calcium

Calcium absorption occurs mainly in the duodenum and proximal jejunum and is facilitated by vitamin D in an acid environment. Thus, any BS that bypass the first part of the intestine, reduces gastric acid production and lowers vitamin D levels is often associated with reduced calcium absorption [15]. The prevalence of calcium deficiency post LGG and RYGB is 3.9% and 4.3 respectively [37]. Low calcium level may affect bone mineralization, therefore, should be supplemented routinely post BS [8].

3.6 Trace elements

Although most of the literature focuses on calcium and iron, deficiencies of other essential minerals such, zinc, copper, and selenium have been reported in bariatric patients [10]. These essential minerals act as enzymatic cofactors in several biochemical pathways, and therefore, their deficiency could cause variable clinical manifestations that involve neurological, cardiac and gastrointestinal systems. Mineral deficiencies are more common after BPD and RYGB [6].

3.6.1 Zinc

Zinc is absorbed by the small intestine and hence BS such RYGB or BPD/DS which partially exclude nutrient from the small bowel, can cause zinc malabsorption [16]. The prevalence of zinc deficiency is 23.9% after LSG [38]. Moderate zinc deficiency presents with hypogeusia, hyposmia, anorexia, eczema, somnolence, and reduced dark adaptation, whereas severe forms are associated with acrodermatitis enteropathica, bullous or pustular dermatitis, diarrhea, balding, mental abnormalities including depression, and recurrent infections due to impaired immune function [16].

3.6.2 Copper

Copper functions as a cofactor in many enzymatic reactions that are vital for the hematologic, vascular, skeletal, antioxidant, and neurologic systems [39]. It is absorbed mainly in the stomach and proximal duodenum. Copper deficiency is rare and underrecognized. More recently, it has been reported after malabsorptive procedures [39]. Symptoms of copper deficiency are often similar to symptoms of vitamin B12 deficiency (hematological and neurological problems). Peripheral neuropathy, myeloneuropathy with spastic ataxic gait have been reported after BS [40]. Recently, a case of severe pancytopenia with refractory anemia secondary to copper deficiency has been observed after BS [39]. In this case, administration of intravenous copper resulted in dramatic clinical improvement [39].

3.6.3 Selenium

Selenium is absorbed in the duodenum and proximal jejunum and it is an essential element that provides an important part of the multifunctional selenoproteins that are important for health [41]. Selenium deficiency has been associated with cardiomyopathy, immune system dysfunction and infertility in men. Since RYGB results in the bypass of the duodenum and upper jejunum, micronutrient deficiencies such as selenium are common after this procedure. The prevalence of selenium deficiency post LSG is 7.1% and post RYGB is 3.8% [26]. A case report described a 40 year-old woman that presented with symptoms of heart failure nine months after RYGB which was confirmed by echocardiography and cardiac markers [42]. The patient was diagnosed with selenium-deficient cardiomyopathy, and she had complete resolution of her symptoms after 3 months of oral selenium [42].

4. Protein malnutrition post bariatric surgery

Protein malnutrition remains the most serious macronutrient complication associated with malabsorptive surgical procedures. It can occur in up to 15% of patients after BPD/DS [43]. Studies reported that 3·0–18·5% of BPD/DS patients required reversal of their procedure because of protein malnutrition or excessive weight loss, or both [44]. Protein malnutrition can also occur after RYGB specially when the Roux limb exceeds 150 cm, where the reported prevalence is 9% at 2 years after surgery [43]; however protein malnutrition rarely necessitates reversal or conversion of a RYGB. It is also less common after LSG and LAGB, and in such cases it is likely due to maladaptive eating behaviors after surgery, especially in patients who avoid protein food sources or have protracted vomiting [6]. The clinical presentation of protein malnutrition includes edema, fatigue, skin, hair, and nail problems [6]. Because protein level often remains in the normal range until late, monitoring the serum albumin concentration is more useful for the assessment of the protein nutritional status. Patients with severe protein malnutrition should be treated with protein supplements that are rich in branch-chain amino acids and, in severe cases enteral feeding is recommended [6]. For prevention of protein malnutrition, an average daily protein intake of 60–120 g (1.1 g/kg of ideal body weight) is required and should be increased by 30% for patients post BPD/BD [16].

5. Complications of micro nutritional deficiencies post bariatric surgery

5.1 Anemia

Anemia is common after BS. The prevalence of macrocytic and microcytic anemia is 52% post LSG, 64% post RYGB and 39% after biliopancreatic diversion [45]. Patients with mild anemia post BS are likely to be asymptomatic; however, when the anemia worsens, patients could present with symptoms, such as fatigue, pallor, and dyspnea on exertion [6]. Post-bariatric anemia is in most cases due to iron deficiency, along with vitamin B12 deficiency as a secondary cause. Other causes of nutritional anemias after malabsorptive BS includes folate, protein, copper, selenium, and zinc deficiencies. Therefore, these factors should be evaluated if routine screening for iron-deficiency anemia is negative [10].

5.2 Neurological complications

Neurological complications may occur after BS. They have attracted attention because of their diversity, complexity and potentially devastating effects [46]. Different patterns of complications can be observed according to the time of presentation. For instance, at an early stage, immediate peripherical nerve injury, Wernicke's encephalopathy, and polyradiculoneuropathy are the most frequent. Late complications may appear after years, and include optic neuropathy, myelopathy, and peripherical neuropathy [47]. The prevalence of neurological events after BS is difficult to determine. A cross-sectional study reported a rate of 3% among 451 patients who underwent BS [48]. Axonal polyneuropathy was the most frequent neurological complication, but cases of Wernicke syndrome, vitamin B12 deficiency, Guillain-Barre syndrome and copper deficiency were also identified [44]. The majority of patients (93.3%) had full recovery from the neurological signs and symptoms [49]. In another retrospective study involving 592 post LSG patients, only 1.18% were found to have neurological complications [50]. In this cohort, all the patients had decrease in oral intake and rapid weight loss, with a mean weight loss of 35 kg three months after LSG suggesting that this could be the predisposing cause [50]. All patients were treated for neuropathy secondary to vitamin B1 deficiency and had significant improvement and/or resolution of their symptoms. [50]. A recent study showed that among 61 patients post RYGB and LAGB, 11.4% developed some signs of polyneuropathy, that eventually disappeared at 24 months. The most common manifestations were paresthesia and muscle weakness [51]. The majority of neurological complications post BS is attributed to vitamin and micronutrient deficiencies such as vitamins B12, B6, E, thiamine, folate and copper [23, 47, 46]. It is imperative to note that failure of diagnosis and the delay in the management of these complications can lead to irreversible neurological deficits. However, many of these complications can be prevented with regular follow-ups, routine screening of micronutrients, and nutritional supplementation where a deficiency is identified.

5.3 Metabolic bone disease

The bone mineral density rapidly decreases initially after BS, which reflects a skeletal adaptation to a lower body weight. Bone loss however, continues even after weight loss has stopped [52]. This is likely due to the lower calcium absorption and vitamin D deficiency causing secondary hyperparathyroidism [53]. The prevalence of secondary hyperparathyroidism has been shown to increase progressively with time from 35.4% at 1 year after BS to 63.3% at 5 years after surgery [54]. Patients who underwent a single anastomosis gastric bypass had the highest prevalence of secondary hyperparathyroidism (73.6%) followed by RYGB (56.6%), gastric banding (38.5%), and sleeve gastrectomy (41.7%) at 5 years after surgery [54]. The decrease in bone density may predispose patients to the risk of fractures especially with malabsorptive procedures. However, data on the incidence of fractures post BS remain controversial, with some studies suggesting an increased risk of fractures (non-vertebral fractures, especially in the upper limbs) and others showing no increased risk [55–57]. For instance, one study reported a significantly increased number of fractures only after biliopancreatic diversion (adjusted relative risk 1·60, 95% CI 1·25–2·03; $p < 0·001$, 56]. Others found that 60% of LAGB and 29% of RYGB patients had increased risk of fractures 3–4 years after surgery [55]. Future long-term studies are required to assess the effect of BS on bone health.

Evaluation of patients for metabolic bone disease after BS may include serum parathyroid hormone, total calcium, phosphorus, 25-hydroxyvitamin D, and

24-hour urine calcium levels [10]. In post-bariatric patients with established osteoporosis, pharmacologic treatment with bisphosphonates may be considered. Before starting bisphosphonate treatment, vitamin D deficiency needs to be fully corrected in order to avoid severe hypocalcaemia, hypophosphatemia, and osteomalacia. In these cases, intravenous form of bisphosphonates should be used (zoledronic acid, 5 mg once a year, or ibandronate, 3 mg every 3 months) for better absorption and to avoid potential anastomotic ulceration with orally administered bisphosphonates [10]. More research is needed to examine the effectiveness of both intravenous and oral bisphosphonates in improving bone mineralization [15].

6. Guidelines for nutritional management post bariatric surgery

Recently, updated guidelines for post-operative nutritional and metabolic support of patients post bariatric surgery were published by the American Association of Clinical Endocrinologists in collaboration with multiple societies [10].

- The follow-up should be scheduled depending on the bariatric procedure performed.
    - For LAGB, it should monthly for the first year and then annually
    - For LSG, it is recommended at 1, 3, 6, 12 months and then annually
    - For RYGB, the recommended follow up is at 1, 3, 6, 12 months and biannually or annually thereafter
    - For BPD/DS and other malabsorptive procedure, the recommended follow up is at 1, 3, 6 months and biannual thereafter.
- Routine metabolic and nutritional monitoring is recommended after all bariatric procedures. This includes:
    - Complete metabolic panel, complete blood count with each visit
    - Iron studies at baseline and after BS as needed
    - B12 annually then every 3–6 months for all type of BS (measurement of methylmalonic acid and homocysteine level are optional)
    - Folic acid level (measurement of red blood cell folic acid level is optional), 25-vitamin D and intact parathyroid hormone (PTH) post RYGB and BPD/DS
    - Vitamin A (initially and every 6–12 months thereafter) for BPD/DS and it is optional for RYGB
    - Copper/ceruloplasmin, zinc, selenium evaluation after malabsorptive bariatric surgical procedures (RYGB and BPD/DS) at least annually, or with symptoms of deficiency
    - Thiamine evaluation in symptomatic patients

- Dual-energy X-ray absorptiometry for bone density at 2 years: for RYGB and BPD/DS.

- The recommended micronutrients supplementations post bariatric surgery to prevent nutritional deficiencies include [10]:

    - Two adult multivitamins plus minerals (each containing iron, folic acid, thiamine, zinc, copper; chewable form initially then tablets).

    - Vitamin B12 (Cobalamin): 350–1000 μg dose can be administrated orally (disintegrating tablet, sublingual, or liquid), nasal spray or parenteral (1000 μg monthly intramuscular or subcutaneous).

    - Iron: 18–60 mg of elemental iron daily included in the multivitamins and additional supplements can be added if required.

    - Vitamin D: at least 2000–3000 international units of vitamin D (titrated to therapeutic 25-hydroxyvitamin D levels >30 ng/mL)

    - Elemental calcium: appropriate dose of daily calcium varies by bariatric procedure. About 200–1500 mg daily for LAGB, LSG and RYGB, and 1800–2400 mg daily for or BPD/DS. Calcium citrate is preferred than calcium carbonate because it is better absorbed in the absence of gastric acid.

Commercial products that are used for micronutrient supplementation after BS need to be discussed with a healthcare professional familiar with dietary supplements, since many products are adulterated and/or mislabeled [10].

7. Preventive strategies of nutritional deficiencies

Since increased adherence with follow-up is associated with improved outcomes, various strategies should be implemented to minimize attrition. Addressing the problem of non-adherence in BS will require the support of qualified healthcare professionals [10, 15]. Multidisciplinary teams with strong communication skills and the involvement of behavioral health experts assist in identifying and addressing compliance barriers. The following strategies may help to improve adherence in the bariatric patients and prevent nutritional deficiencies:

- Increase patient engagement in after care appointments. The bariatric team can utilize strategies such as frequent calls, reminders letters, flexible scheduling/variety of appointment times, laboratory results, newsletters to provide reinforcement for follow up [58]

- Develop innovative strategies to address barriers to follow-up, such as remotely delivered interventions, smart-phone apps, and follow up video appointments [59]

- The long-term follow-up visits should include screening for micronutrient deficiencies, bone health, and monitoring of nutrition-related diseases. Reinforcing healthy eating habits is also recommended, such as eating slowly, portion control, and meeting protein requirements

- Focus on adherence in the areas that are most critical for patient well-being. For instance, vitamin deficiency can cause serious health problems, including, in rare cases, encephalopathy

- Address barriers and causes of non-compliance with multivitamins supplementation. For example, the most frequent reasons for non-adherence to vitamins, i.e., forgetting, difficulty swallowing or not liking to take pills. These issues can be solved by using pill organizers and electronic reminders which can assist with memory issues. Offering chewable or liquid form of vitamins to will also aid bariatric patients with swallowing difficulty [59]

- The role of the family physician in bariatric post-surgery care is important to consider. However, the nature of their involvement post-surgery care is currently unclear [60]. Greater role clarity and enhanced collaboration between surgeons, general practitioners and patients following surgery is likely to enhance the experience and outcomes for patients and encourage and support the maintenance of postsurgical care [60].

- Patient education before and after surgery plays a key role in the adherence to micronutrient supplementation and improvement of BS outcomes. Patients should be encouraged to become involved in their own care. Lectures and discussions provided by healthcare experts from multiple disciplines in small groups, or individual sessions utilizing both written or web-based delivery should be done to support learning needs of the bariatric patients. Moreover, patient education methods should focus on high-quality, cost-effective, and patient-centered educational programs for bariatric surgery [61].

8. Conclusions

BS is the most effective strategy for the treatment of severe obesity and for the resolution of comorbid medical conditions. Post-surgery, patients are at increased risk for nutritional deficiencies which may result in serious complications if they are not recognized and treated promptly. Adherence to multivitamins supplementations is important to prevent such deficiencies. Multidisciplinary approach with close monitoring is the key for the long-term success after bariatric surgery.

Conflict of interest

The authors declare no conflict of interest.

Acronyms and abbreviations

BS	bariatric surgery
LAGB	gastric banding
LSG	laparoscopic sleeve gastrectomy
RYGB	Roux en Y gastric bypass
OAGB	one-anastomosis gastric bypass
SADI-S	single anastomosis duodeno–ileal bypass with sleeve gastrectomy
BPD/DS	biliopancreatic diversion with duodenal switch

Author details

Wahiba Elhag[1*] and Walid El Ansari[2,3,4]

1 Department of Bariatric Surgery/Bariatric Medicine, Hamad General Hospital, 3050, Doha, Qatar

2 Department of Surgery, Hamad General Hospital, 3050, Doha, Qatar

3 College of Medicine, Qatar University, Doha, Qatar

4 Schools of Health and Education, University of Skovde, Skövde, Sweden

*Address all correspondence to: welansari9@gmail.com

References

[1] Schauer PR, Bhatt DL, Kirwan JP, et al. Bariatric surgery versus intensive medical therapy for diabetes - 5-year outcomes. The New England Journal of Medicine. 2017;**376**:641-651

[2] Elgenaied I, El Ansari W, Elsherif MA, Abdulrazzaq S, Qabbani AS, Elhag W. Factors associated with complete and partial remission, improvement, or unchanged diabetes status of obese adults 1 year after sleeve gastrectomy. Surg Obes Relat Dis Off J Am Soc Bariatr Surg. 2020

[3] Gregory DM, Twells LK, Lester KK, et al. Preoperative and postoperative assessments of biochemical parameters in patients with severe obesity undergoing laparoscopic sleeve gastrectomy. Obesity Surgery. 2018;**28**:2261-2271

[4] van Rutte PWJ, Aarts EO, Smulders JF, Nienhuijs SW. Nutrient deficiencies before and after sleeve gastrectomy. Obesity Surgery. 2014;**24**:1639-1646

[5] Wolf E, Utech M, Stehle P, Büsing M, Stoffel-Wagner B, Ellinger S. Preoperative micronutrient status in morbidly obese patients before undergoing bariatric surgery: Results of a cross-sectional study. Surg Obes Relat Dis Off J Am Soc Bariatr Surg. 2015;**11**:1157-1163

[6] Lupoli R, Lembo E, Saldalamacchia G, Avola CK, Angrisani L, Capaldo B. Bariatric surgery and long-term nutritional issues. World Journal of Diabetes. 2017;**8**:464-474

[7] Sánchez A, Rojas P, Basfi-fer K, et al. Micronutrient deficiencies in morbidly obese women prior to bariatric surgery. Obesity Surgery. 2016;**26**:361-368

[8] Guan B, Yang J, Chen Y, Yang W, Wang C. Nutritional deficiencies in Chinese patients undergoing gastric bypass and sleeve gastrectomy: Prevalence and predictors. Obesity Surgery. 2018;**28**:2727-2736

[9] Martínez-Ortega AJ, Olveira G, Pereira-Cunill JL, et al. Recommendations Based on Evidence by the Andalusian Group for Nutrition Reflection and Investigation (GARIN) for the Pre- and Postoperative Management of Patients Undergoing Obesity Surgery. Nutrients. 2020;12. Jul 6. doi: 10.3390/nu12072002

[10] Mechanick JI, Apovian C, Brethauer S, et al. Clinical practice guidelines for the perioperative nutrition, metabolic, and nonsurgical support of patients undergoing bariatric procedures - 2019 update: cosponsored by American Association of Clinical Endocrinologists/ American College of Endocrinology, The Obesity Society, American Society for Metabolic & Bariatric Surgery, Obesity Medicine Association, and American Society of Anesthesiologists. Surg Obes Relat Dis Off J Am Soc Bariatr Surg. 2020;**16**:175-247.

[11] Thereaux J, Lesuffleur T, Païta M, et al. Long-term follow-up after bariatric surgery in a national cohort. The British Journal of Surgery. 2017;**104**:1362-1371

[12] Modi AC, Zeller MH, Xanthakos SA, Jenkins TM, Inge TH. Adherence to vitamin supplementation following adolescent bariatric surgery. Obes Silver Spring Md. 2013;**21**:E190-E195

[13] Mehaffey JH, Mehaffey RL, Mullen MG, et al. Nutrient deficiency 10 years following Roux-en-Y gastric bypass: Who's responsible? Obesity Surgery. 2017;**27**:1131-1136

[14] Allied Health Sciences Section Ad Hoc Nutrition Committee,

Aills L, Blankenship J, Buffington C, Furtado M, Parrott J. ASMBS Allied Health Nutritional Guidelines for the Surgical Weight Loss Patient. Surg Obes Relat Dis Off J Am Soc Bariatr Surg. 2008;**4**:S73-108.

[15] Busetto L, Dicker D, Azran C, et al. Obesity Management Task Force of the European Association for the Study of Obesity Released "Practical Recommendations for the Post-Bariatric Surgery Medical Management." Obesity Surgery 2018;**28**:2117-2121.

[16] Mingrone G, Bornstein S, Le Roux CW. Optimisation of follow-up after metabolic surgery. The Lancet Diabetes and Endocrinology. 2018;**6**:487-499

[17] Oudman E, Wijnia JW, van Dam M, Biter LU, Postma A. Preventing Wernicke encephalopathy after bariatric surgery. Obesity Surgery. 2018;**28**:2060-2068

[18] Hamilton LA, Darby SH, Hamilton AJ, Wilkerson MH, Morgan KA. Case report of Wernicke's encephalopathy after sleeve gastrectomy. Nutr Clin Pract Off Publ Am Soc Parenter Enter Nutr. 2018;**33**:510-514

[19] Loh Y, Watson WD, Verma A, Chang ST, Stocker DJ, Labutta RJ. Acute Wernicke's encephalopathy following bariatric surgery: Clinical course and MRI correlation. Obesity Surgery. 2004;**14**:129-132

[20] Negri M, Macerola N, Mancarella FA, et al. A late onset of Wernicke-Korsakoff encephalopathy after biliopancreatic diversion: A case report. Obesity Surgery. 2019;**29**:2309-2311

[21] Boateng AA, Sriram K, Meguid MM, Crook M. Refeeding syndrome: Treatment considerations based on collective analysis of literature case reports. Nutr Burbank Los Angel Cty Calif. 2010;**26**:156-167

[22] Sechi G, Serra A. Wernicke's encephalopathy: New clinical settings and recent advances in diagnosis and management. Lancet Neurology. 2007;**6**:442-455

[23] Becker DA, Ingala EE, Martinez-Lage M, Price RS, Galetta SL. Dry beriberi and Wernicke's encephalopathy following gastric lap band surgery. J Clin Neurosci Off J Neurosurg Soc Australas. 2012;**19**:1050-1052

[24] Damms-Machado A, Friedrich A, Kramer KM, et al. Pre- and postoperative nutritional deficiencies in obese patients undergoing laparoscopic sleeve gastrectomy. Obesity Surgery. 2012;**22**:881-889

[25] Mechanick JI, Kushner RF, Sugerman HJ, et al. American Association of Clinical Endocrinologists, The Obesity Society, and American Society for Metabolic & Bariatric Surgery medical guidelines for clinical practice for the perioperative nutritional, metabolic, and nonsurgical support of the bariatric surgery patient. Obes Silver Spring Md. 2009;**17** Suppl 1:S1-70, v.

[26] Vinolas H, Barnetche T, Ferrandi G, et al. Oral hydration, food intake, and nutritional status before and after bariatric surgery. Obesity Surgery. 2019;**29**:2896-2903

[27] Jans G, Matthys C, Bogaerts A, et al. Maternal micronutrient deficiencies and related adverse neonatal outcomes after bariatric surgery: A systematic review. Adv Nutr Bethesda Md. 2015;**6**:420-429

[28] Cruz S, Machado S, Cruz S, Pereira S, Saboya C, Ramalho A. Comparative study of the nutritional status of vitamin a in pregnant women and in women who became pregnant or did not after Roux-en-Y gastric bypass. Nutrición Hospitalaria. 2018;**35**:421-427

[29] Alejo Ramos M, Cano Rodríguez IM, Urioste Fondo AM, et al. Secondary hyperparathyroidism in patients with biliopancreatic diversion after 10 years of follow-up, and relationship with vitamin D and serum calcium. Obesity Surgery. 2019;**29**:999-1006

[30] Parrott J, Frank L, Rabena R, Craggs-Dino L, Isom KA, Greiman L. American Society for Metabolic and Bariatric Surgery Integrated Health Nutritional Guidelines for the surgical weight loss patient 2016 update: Micronutrients. Surg Obes Relat Dis Off J Am Soc Bariatr Surg. 2017;**13**:727-741

[31] Enochs P, Bull J, Surve A, et al. Comparative analysis of the single-anastomosis duodenal-ileal bypass with sleeve gastrectomy (SADI-S) to established bariatric procedures: An assessment of 2-year postoperative data illustrating weight loss, type 2 diabetes, and nutritional status in a single US center. Surg Obes Relat Dis. Elsevier. 2020;**16**:24-33

[32] Van Mieghem T, Van Schoubroeck D, Depiere M, Debeer A, Hanssens M. Fetal cerebral hemorrhage caused by vitamin K deficiency after complicated bariatric surgery. Obstetrics and Gynecology. 2008;**112**:434-436

[33] Cuesta M, Pelaz L, Pérez C, et al. Fat-soluble vitamin deficiencies after bariatric surgery could be misleading if they are not appropriately adjusted. Nutrición Hospitalaria. 2014;**30**:118-123

[34] Obinwanne KM, Fredrickson KA, Mathiason MA, Kallies KJ, Farnen JP, Kothari SN. Incidence, treatment, and outcomes of iron deficiency after laparoscopic Roux-en-Y gastric bypass: A 10-year analysis. Journal of the American College of Surgeons. 2014;**218**:246-252

[35] Gloy VL, Briel M, Bhatt DL, Kashyap SR, et al. Bariatric surgery versus non-surgical treatment for obesity: A systematic review and meta-analysis of randomised controlled trials. BMJ. 2013;**347**:f5934

[36] Gowanlock Z, Lezhanska A, Conroy M, et al. Iron deficiency following bariatric surgery: A retrospective cohort study. Blood Advances. 2020;**4**:3639-3647

[37] Antoniewicz A, Kalinowski P, Kotulecka KJ, et al. Nutritional deficiencies in patients after Roux-en-Y gastric bypass and sleeve gastrectomy during 12-month follow-up. Obesity Surgery. 2019;**29**:3277-3284

[38] Belfiore A, Cataldi M, Minichini L, et al. Short-term changes in body composition and response to micronutrient supplementation after laparoscopic sleeve gastrectomy. Obesity Surgery. 2015;**25**:2344-2351

[39] Abusabeib A, El Ansari W, Elhag W. First case report of acquired copper deficiency following Revisional single anastomosis Duodeno-ileal bypass with sleeve gastrectomy (SADI-S) leading to severe pancytopenia with refractory anemia. Obesity Surgery. 2020:1-4. DOI: 10.1007/s11695-020-04916-3

[40] Robinson SD, Cooper B, Leday TV. Copper deficiency (hypocupremia) and pancytopenia late after gastric bypass surgery. Proc Bayl Univ Med Cent. 2013;**26**:382-386

[41] Hassan Zadeh M, Mohammadi Farsani G, Zamaninour N. Selenium status after Roux-en-Y gastric bypass: Interventions and recommendations. Obesity Surgery. 2019;**29**:3743-3748

[42] Massoure P-L, Camus O, Fourcade L, Simon F. Bilateral leg oedema after bariatric surgery: A selenium-deficient cardiomyopathy. Obesity Research & Clinical Practice. 2017;**11**:622-626

[43] Suárez Llanos JP, Fuentes Ferrer M, Alvarez-Sala-Walther L, et al. PROTEIN MALNUTRITION INCIDENCE COMPARISON AFTER GASTRIC BYPASS VERSUS BILIOPANCREATIC DIVERSION. Nutrición Hospitalaria. 2015;**32**:80-86

[44] Bolckmans R, Himpens J. Long-term (>10 Yrs) outcome of the laparoscopic biliopancreatic diversion with duodenal switch. Annals of Surgery. 2016;**264**:1029-1037

[45] Mingrone G, Bornstein S, Le Roux CW. Optimisation of follow-up after metabolic surgery. The Lancet Diabetes and Endocrinology. 2018;**6**:487-499

[46] Zafar A, Khatri IA. An overview of complications affecting the central nervous system following bariatric surgery. Neurosci Riyadh Saudi Arab. 2018;**23**:4-12

[47] Landais A. Neurological complications of bariatric surgery. Obesity Surgery. 2014;**24**:1800-1807

[48] Algahtani HA, Khan AS, Khan MA, Aldarmahi AA, Lodhi Y. Neurological complications of bariatric surgery. Neurosci Riyadh Saudi Arab. 2016;**21**:241-245

[49] Alqahtani A, Elahmedi M, Qahtani ARA. Laparoscopic sleeve gastrectomy in children younger than 14 years: Refuting the concerns. Annals of Surgery. 2016;**263**:312-319

[50] Tabbara M, Carandina S, Bossi M, Polliand C, Genser L, Barrat C. Rare neurological complications after sleeve gastrectomy. Obesity Surgery. 2016;**26**:2843-2848

[51] Riccò M, Rapacchi C, Romboli A, et al. Peripheral neuropathies after bariatric surgery. Preliminary results from a single-Centre prospective study in northern Italy. Acta Bio-Medica Atenei Parm. 2019;**90**:259-265

[52] Shanbhogue VV, Støving RK, Frederiksen KH, et al. Bone structural changes after gastric bypass surgery evaluated by HR-pQCT: A two-year longitudinal study. European Journal of Endocrinology. 2017;**176**:685-693

[53] Costa TL, Paganotto M, Radominski RB, Kulak CM, Borba VC. Calcium metabolism, vitamin D and bone mineral density after bariatric surgery. Osteoporosis International. 2015;**26**:757-764

[54] Wei J-H, Lee W-J, Chong K, et al. High incidence of secondary hyperparathyroidism in bariatric patients: Comparing different procedures. Obesity Surgery. 2018;**28**:798-804

[55] Lalmohamed A, de Vries F, Bazelier MT, Cooper A, van Staa T-P, Cooper C, et al. Risk of fracture after bariatric surgery in the United Kingdom: Population based, retrospective cohort study. BMJ. 2012;**345**:e5085

[56] Rousseau C, Jean S, Gamache P, et al. Change in fracture risk and fracture pattern after bariatric surgery: Nested case-control study. BMJ. 2016;**354**:i3794

[57] Zhang Q, Chen Y, Li J, et al. A meta-analysis of the effects of bariatric surgery on fracture risk. Obes Rev Off J Int Assoc Study Obes. 2018;**19**:728-736

[58] Gourash WF, Ebel F, Lancaster K, et al. Longitudinal assessment of bariatric surgery (LABS): Retention strategy and results at 24 months. Surg Obes Relat Dis Off J Am Soc Bariatr Surg. 2013;**9**:514-519

[59] Hood MM, Corsica J, Bradley L, Wilson R, Chirinos DA, Vivo A. Managing severe obesity:

Understanding and improving treatment adherence in bariatric surgery. Journal of Behavioral Medicine. 2016;**39**:1092-1103

[60] Jose K, Venn A, Nelson M, Howes F, Wilkinson S, Ezzy D. A qualitative study of the role of Australian general practitioners in the surgical management of obesity. Clin Obes. 2017;**7**:231-238

[61] Groller KD. Systematic review of patient education practices in weight loss surgery. Surg Obes Relat Dis Off J Am Soc Bariatr Surg. 2017;**13**:1072-1085

Chapter 5

Bariatric Surgery—from the Non-surgical Approach to the Post-Surgery Individual Care: Role of Endoscopy in Bariatric Therapy

Dörte Wichmann, Dietmar Stüker, Ulrich Schweizer, Alfred Königsrainer and Rami Archid

Abstract

Obesity is the underlying constant for the development of the most common modern diseases such as insulin resistance, high blood pressure, lipid metabolism disorders, non-alcoholic steatohepatitis (fatty liver), joint problems and various malignancies. The role of endoscopic diagnostic and therapy in obese patients is highlighted in this chapter. In this chapter all devices and methods used in flexible endoscopy for diagnostic and treatment in obese patients are introduced. Role of endoscopy is presented in three parts: in preoperative setting, in post-operative complication management and instead of surgery as endoscopic bariatric therapy. If possible presentation of the effectiveness is compiled with study data. Finally, the interaction between endoscopy and surgery in the treatment of obesity is complex, essential and promising. Endoscopy is indispensable in preoperative preparation, as a primary therapeutic approach, and also in the detection and treatment of acute complications and long-term complications of obesity surgery.

Keywords: endoscopic bariatric therapy, endoscopic complication management

1. Introduction

The annual number of obesity surgery and metabolic interventions increased worldwide significantly and the continued pressure to provide ambulatory surgery, endoluminal, and transgastric therapy has the potential to effect major changes in the way obesity is treated. Covering the "market demand" simply by further increasing the number of operations seems illusory if the prevalence of obesity is still rising. Endoluminal surgery is defined as surgery performed entirely within the lumen of the gastrointestinal tract using flexible endoscopy.

The interaction between endoscopy and surgery in the treatment of obesity is complex, essential and promising. Endoscopy is indispensable in preoperative preparation, as a primary therapeutic approach, and also in the detection and treatment of acute complications and long-term complications of obesity surgery.

The currently established and developing endoscopic procedures for bariatric therapy will be presented in this chapter. Division into pre-operative endoscopy,

IntechOpen

endoscopic bariatric therapy (EBT) and post-surgical endoscopy for early and late complications was made.

2. Preoperative setting: diagnostic esophago-gastro-duodenoscopy

In "The clinical practice guidelines of the EAES on bariatric surgery: update 2020" the indication of a pre-operative EGD has been approved [1]. Clinically significant gastrointestinal (GI) symptoms should be evaluated before bariatric procedures with imaging studies, upper GI series, or endoscopy. All patients who where enrolled for a sleeve gastrectomy have to be examined with a gastroscopy for presence of hiatal hernia and esophageal reflux. Endoscopists have to look for signs of GERD. This diagnosis is a contraindication for a sleeve gastrectomy. Presence of hiatal hernia is also important from the surgical point of view, as it also needs to be repaired while bariatric surgery. In the diagnostic gastroscopy Helicobacter-pylorii diagnosis has to been established. Recent studies illustrate a relationship of Helicobacter pylori with the occurrence of marginal ulcers postoperatively especially following RYGB.

3. Endoscopic bariatric therapy

Primary endoscopic obesity therapy has now been given the proper name "bariatric endoscopy" or "endoscopic bariatric therapy". This illustrates the relevance of endoscopy for the treatment of obese patients. EBT currently includes six different mechanisms:

1. Space occupying
2. Endoscopic gastroplasty
3. Aspiration
4. Malabsorption
5. Endoscopic bypass
6. Others

In **Table 1** we present an overview of all endoscopic therapeutic concepts with available correlated EWL is presented.

For the completeness of the review, the swallow balloons Elipse™ and OBALLON™ are mentioned at this point. However, they do not require endoscopic control or filling and are therefore not considered further in this review.

EAES and IFSO guidelines recommend consultation on surgical or endoscopic bariatric therapy based on initial weight, previous eating habits, expected weight loss, patient-related risk stratification (pre-existing conditions, compliance) and local availability of surgical and/or endoscopic bariatric surgery experts EAES 2020 [1, 10]. The choice of bariatric intervention should be based on the consensus of a supervising, interdisciplinary board of experts, whose members are from the fields of surgery, nutritional medicine, endocrinology and psychology, and the fully informed patient.

Mechanism	Product	Time	EWL
1. Space occupying	1.1 Spatz3 one-year-balloon	12 months	67.4% [2, 3]
	1.2 ReShape™ Dual Balloon	6 months	29.9% [4]
	1.3 ORBERA™ Intragastric Balloon	6 months	25.44% [5]
	1.4 Transpyloric shuttle™	6 months	30.9% [6]
	1.5 Heliosphere bag	6 months	31.87% [7, 8]
2. Endoscopic gastroplasty	2.1 POSE™	permanent	49.4% [9]
	2.2 ESG (Endoscopic Sleeve gastrectomy, Apollo OverStitch)	permanent	61.84-68.3% [10–12]
	2.3 RESTORe (EndoCinch)	permanent	58.1% [13, 14]
	2.4 TOGA (transorale gastroplasty)	permanent	38.7% [15]
	2.5 TERIS (trans-oral endoscopic restrictive implant system)	6 months	30.1% [16]
	2.6 ACE-Stapler	permanent	34.9% [13, 17]
	2.7 Endomina System	permanent	41% [13]
3. Aspiration	Aspire Assist®	6-24 months	31.5% [18]
4. Malabsorption	4.1 EndoBarrier® (Duodeno-Jejunale liner)	12 months	35.3% [13, 19]
	4.2 ValenTx™ (Gastro-Duodeno-Jejunale Liner)	12 months	39.7% [20]
	4.3 DMR (endoscopic hydrothermal Duodenal Mucosal Resurfacing)	permanent	-
5. Endoscopic Bypass	Incisionless Magnetic Anastamosis System (IMAS)	permanent	40.2% [21]
6. Others	6.1 Full Sense	-	-
	6.2 Satisphere	-	-

Table 1.
Mechanisms of endoscopic bariatric treatment, products and procedures are listed with mean EWL% after 12 months if available.

In **Figure 1** following mechanisms and products are illustrated in a sketch:
A = Orbera Intragastric Balloon
B = ReShape Duo Intragastric Balloon
C = TransPyloric Shuttle
D = POSE™
E = ESG with Apollo OverStitch™
F = Endomina
G = Aspire Assist
H = EndoBarrier
I = Satisphere device

3.1 Space occupying

The common gastric balloons are well accepted. Besides the expected nausea and belching, possible gastric ulcerations and perforations should be discussed with the patients.

All endoscopic, bariatric mechanisms that have a timely limit should be combined with an intensive nutritional, medical and psychological therapy. Obesity is a chronic disease, so there is always the risk of a "yo-yo" effect after removal of the space occupying device in such procedures. This development must be discussed with the patient.

The time-limited procedures are particularly suitable with a step-by-step concept prior to bariatric surgery.

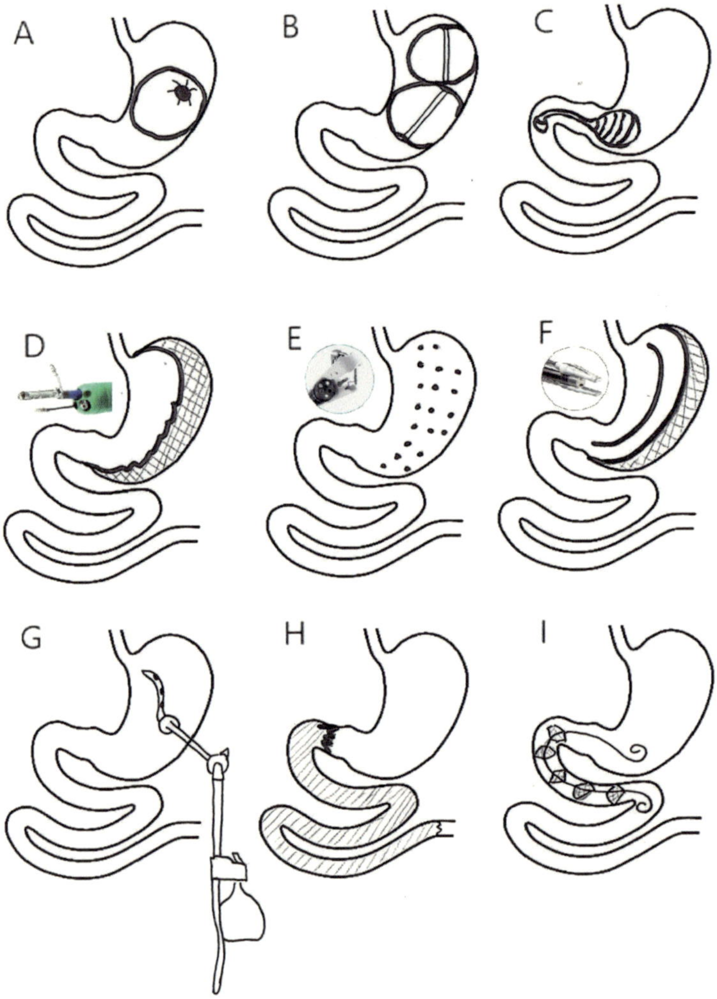

Figure 1.
Relevant techniques and devices of EBT are sketchily presented. A) Orbera Intragastric balloon. B) Reshape duo Intragastric balloon. C) Transpyloric shuttle-device. D) POSE™ operating platform with fundal accomodation. E) Endoscopic gastric sleeve with the OverStitch™-device. F) Endomina-suturing-system. G) Aspire assist-device. H) Endobarrier duodeno-jejunal bypass liner. I) SatiSphere-device.

3.1.1 Spatz3

The Spatz3 (Spatz FGIA, Great Neck, NY, USA) intragastric balloon is the only space occupying system for using a time of 12 months. The balloon is placed endoscopically and filled with 400-750 ml saline and methylene blue.

Results: Usuy and Brooks reported 2018 about 165 patients with implanted Spatz3 balloons in two centers. Mean EWL after one year was 67.4% [3].

Complications: Complications were nausea (89–92%), vomiting (21–71%), and abdominal pain (22–24%). Five patients developed gastric ulcers, one gastric perforation occurred at week 17 after implantation.

3.2 ReShape duo intragastric balloon

The ReShape IGB (Reshape, San Clemente, CA, USA) device contains of two silicone balloons attached to each other by a flexible tube. It is inserted and retrieved endoscopically. Device is placed for 6 months. The ReShape Duo is filled with 900 mL of saline solution (450 mL to each balloon). Each balloon has independent channels to prevent deflation of the other balloon if one leaks.

Results: In a seven-center study of Agnihotri and colleagues 202 patients were enrolled. EWL after 6 months was 29.9% [4]. In the REDUCE pivotal trial, including 326 patients, EWL was 25.1% in the Reshape arm compared to 11.3% in the sham arm [22].

Complications: Most common SAEs were nausea, vomiting, and abdominal pain that generally resolved after 1 week. The gastric ulceration rate was 0.9%.

3.3 Orbera

The Orbera (Apollo Endosurgery, Austin, TX, USA) is a single, spherical balloon composed of silicone previously known as the BioEnterics Intragastric Balloon (BIB; Allergan, Irvine, California, USA). The balloon filling volume ranges between 400 and 700 mL of saline.

Results: Courcoulas and colleagues [23] reported in a multicenter, randomized, comparative study about 137 patients with implanted Orbera balloon. Mean EWL after 9 months was 26.5%.

Complications: Early removal of the IGB occurred in 18.75% of patients. The most common adverse events were pain and nausea [23]. Reported SAEs with this balloon were rare, and consisted of migration in 1.4% of patients and gastric perforation in 0.1% [24].

3.4 TransPyloric shuttle

The TransPyloric Shuttle (BAROnova Inc. Goleta, CA) consists of a spherical silicone bulb attached to a smaller silicone bulb by a flexible tether. Intermitted occlusion of the gastric antrum is reached by the larger bulb when the smaller bulb entering the duodenum with peristalsis.

Results: A randomized clinical trial showed a mean EWL of 30.9% at 12 months follow-up [6].

Complications: Premature balloon removal occurred in 22.7% (46/203) of the cases. SAEs were rare (2.8%) and included: esophageal rupture, device impaction, upper abdominal pain, gastric ulcer, vomiting, pneumothorax. Premature balloon removal occurred in 22.7% (46/203) of the cases.

3.5 Heliosphere bag

The Heliosphere BAG is filled with 950 mL of air rather than fluid. Balloons were implanted for six months.

Results: Lecumberri and colleagues reported about 82 patients with a EWL of 31.87% six months after insertion [8].

Complications: The Heliosphere BAG deflated and passed spontaneously in 2 cases (3%). De Castro et al. [25] described 2013 a comparative, prospective study of 91 patients: Orbera balloon (73 patients) with Heliosphere BAG (18 patients, mean BMI 45.2 kg/m^2). In this study balloon extraction was difficult in 8 cases, and a rigid esophagoscope as required in 4 cases; laparoscopic surgery was required to remove BAG in 1 case. BAG was significantly more likely to result in retrieval complications.

4. Endoscopic gastroplasty, endoscopic sleeve

Endoscopic gastroplasty or sleeve procedures are enjoying increasing popularity. The principle of all the procedures listed is a reduction of the stomach volume by endoluminally placed sutures or clips. The procedures are performed transorally, so that no permanent scars result. By means of a suture/clip machine placed on the endoscope, the stomach is contracted from the intraluminal side and fixed accordingly, thus reducing its lumen. The change in the shape and function of the stomach primarily leads to delayed gastric emptying and thus increased saturation. Weight loss and reduction of the diabetic metabolic state are the result. These procedures have been evaluated for patients with obesity class 1 to 3 and are associated with excellent long-term results.

4.1 POSE™

Primary obesity surgery endoluminal (POSE) uses the incisionless operating platform (IOP; USGI Medical, San Clemente, CA, USA) to create full-thickness plications in the gastric fundus to reduce gastric volume. The Pose procedure targeted the gastric fundal accommodation. In 2020 López-Navada presented the POSE 2 procedure. Using the same devices, the POSE-2 procedure attempts to impair the gastric motility and restrict the gastric volume [26].

Results: Lopez-Navada et al. reported 2015 about 147 patients who underwent POSE procedure and were followed for one year [9]. Mean EWL was 44.9%. In a meta-analysis of Khan et al. with 7 included studies about POSE procedure Mean pooled EWL after 12 months was 44.91% [27].

Complications: Lopez-Navada reported that short-term adverse events included minor bleeding at the suture site, which was managed without incidence. Sullivan et al. [28], one of the included studies of the meta-analysis of Khan et al., reported that 45% of patients had post-procedure abdominal pain requiring pharmacotherapy, and 40% reported nausea and vomiting. For POSE 2 procedure no AEs were reported.

4.2 ESG (endoscopic sleeve gastrectomy) with the Apollo OverStitch™

The Apollo OverStitch™ (Apollo Endosurgery, Austin, TX) is an endoscopic suturing device that applies full-thickness sutures in a variety of patterns. The system attaches to a double-channel endoscope and utilizes a curved needle driver. The OverStitch Sx™ is available for using single working channel endoscopes.

Results: In the meta-analysis of Gys and colleagues from 2019 eight clinical trials (1721 patients, 2014–2019) were included with 6–24 months follow-up. Average pooled EWL at 12 months was 68.3% [12]. In the recent meta-analysis of Singh and colleagues pooled EWL after 12 months was 61.84% [11].

Complications: In the analysis of Gys et al. major adverse events were described in 18 patients: pneumothorax (n = 2), perigastric collection (n = 8), pulmonary embolism (n = 2), intraluminal bleeding (n = 5), and leakage (n = 1). Singh et al. described a pooled incidence of serious adverse events of 2.26%.

4.3 RESTORe with the EndoCinch device

Endoluminal Vertical Gastroplasty (EVG) is performed using the EndoCinch suturing device (C.R. Bard, Inc., Murray Hill, NJ). Since 2004 this device is used to treat obesity. The RESTORe System (Bard/Davol, Warwick, RI) is an updated version of the EndoCinch device. It is capable of deeper tissue acquisition and suture reloading inside the patient. During this procedure, in addition to an anterior to posterior plication in EVG, the greater curvature is also incorporated to mimic LGP.

Results: In 2008, Fogel performed EVG in 64 patients using a continuous running suture along the lesser curvature. No serious adverse events were reported and weight loss at 1 year was 58.1% EWL [14].

Complications: No significant adverse events were seen. Twelve-month endoscopy revealed partial or complete release of plications in 13 of 18 patients.

4.4 TOGA (transorale Gastroplasie)

TOGA (Satiety Inc., Palo Alto, CA) is an endoscopic stapling device first introduced in 2008. TOGA creates a stapled sleeve and a restricted outlet. Similar to VBG, TOGA is associated with decreased ghrelin and increased GLP-1 levels.

Results: A sham-controlled trial including 67 patients showed 52.2% EWL (in patients with BMI < 40) and 41.3% EWL (in those with BMI ≥ 40) after one year [15].

Complications: Two cases of respiratory distress and an asymptomatic pneumoperitoneum from esophageal and gastric perforations that was treated conservatively however were reported.

4.5 TERIS (trans-oral endoscopic restrictive implant system)

TERIS (Barosense, Redwood City, CA) is an endoscopically implanted device introduced by Biertho and colleagues in 2009. A prosthetic diaphragm is placed at the gastric cardia to create a small reservoir with a 10-mm orifice. To anchor the device full thickness plications are used.

Results: In a study including 18 patients (mean BMI 42.1 kg/m^2) Verlaan et al. reported about a median EWL after six month of 30.1% [16].

Complications: Three SAEs occurred, one gastric perforation and two cases of pneumoperitoneum. Because of the poor durability of the system the company decided to discontinue the TERIS system and to further develop the successful parts of it, such as the articulating circular endoscopic (ACE) stapler.

4.6 ACE-stapler (articulating circular endoscopic stapler)

The ACE stapler (Boston Scientific Corporation, Natick, MA) is an endoscopic stapler. This device consist of a head capable of both 360-degree rotation and complete retroflexion. A 5-mm endoscope enables visualization; the device is 16 mm in diameter. This device use vacuum suction to mobilize gastric tissue; firing the stapler creates a full-thickness plication using a 10-mm plastic ring with 8 titanium staples. A defined number of plications is done in the fundus and antrum.

Results: Verlaan et al. [17] reported about 17 patients (BMI 40.2 kg/m^2) et al. reported in a prospective safety and feasibility study of gastric volume reduction. Median EWL was 34.9%.

Complications: The most common adverse event was abdominal pain (7 patients); sore throat, diarrhea, nausea, constipation, and vomiting were also reported. All were self-limited.

4.7 Endomina system

The Endomina suturing system (Endo Tools Therapeutics, SA-ETT, Gosselies, Belgium) is a triangulation platform to perform large plications with transmural sutures and serosa-to-serosa apposition to reduce the gastric volume.

Results: Two studies (62 patients) by Huberty et al. reported 29% EWL at 12 months [29, 30].

Complications: No major adverse events were reported.

5. Aspiration therapy

Nyström et al. [26] reported 2018 in a 4-year analysis on the results of the AspireAssist® system in 201 bariatric patients, including in particular class 2 and 3 obese patients. Using a modified PEG, patients can drain the food pulp and rinse with water 20 minutes after ingestion. This device could reduce the absorption of up to 30% ingested calories after a meal.

Results: EWL and TWL rates of 43.6% and 17.1%respectively were achieved after one year.

Complications: The complication rate corresponds to that of PEG (inflammation of the injection site, peritonitis, buried bumper).

6. Malabsorption

The procedures that lead to a barrier development of duodeno-jejunal or gastro-duodeno-jejunal contact are endoscopic, innovative interpretations of the mode of action of the surgically created gastric bypass. The implantation of a plastic liner into the lumen of these organs can result in good glycaemic control and, in addition, weight reduction. These procedures are named gastrointestinal bypass liners (EndoBarrier®, ValenTx™). They are particularly indicated for patients with poorly adjustable diabetes mellitus type II.

6.1 The EndoBarrier

The EndoBarrier consists of a single use endoscopic system including a liner, delivery system, and retrieval system. A 65 cm teflon covered sleeve is placed into the small bowel and can remain in situ for up to 3–12 months. Endoscopically implementation is done under general anesthesia. Placement of anchor and liner is controlled by endoscopy and fluoroscopic guidance. The anchors at the proximal end of the sleeve looks like a crown, consists of nitinol, which functions as a self-expandable stent. This allows fixation to the duodenal bulb distal to the pylorus, but proximal to the ampulla Vateri. The proximal and distal open liner ensures the passage of chyme from the stomach while bypassing the duodenum. Along the outside of the liner, pancreatic juices and bile will enter from the ampulla Vateri, thereby avoiding contact with gastric contents until these exit the sleeve in the jejunum. The EndoBarrier mimics the malabsorptive effects of the RYGB.

Results: Betzel and colleagues [19] reported 2020 about 44 patients treated with EndoBarrier-Devices. Twenty patients required early removal due to AEs(55%). During dwelling time, body weight decreased significantly (15.9 kg; TBWL 14.6%). HbA1c decreased non-significantly. In total, 68% of the patients experienced at least one AE. Patel et al. [31] 2018 reported about similar results in a multicenter, non-randomized clinical trial with 45 obese patients. Fourteen patients required early removal (24%). Significant reductions in weight, BMI and glycaemic control were observed during the device insertion period.

Complications: The ASGE Bariatric Endoscopy Task Force reported 2015 about an AE rate of 12.66% in 271 implantation [10]. Serious adverse events included migration (4.9%), GI bleeding (3.86%), sleeve obstruction (3.4%), liver abscess (0.126%), cholangitis (0.126%), acute cholecystitis (0.126%), and esophageal perforation(0.126%).

6.2 The ValenTx and its successor

The ValenTx-System is a gastro-duodenal-jejunal liner system which has to be inserted in an endoscopic/laparoscopic rendezvous technique. The system, a 120 cm long fluoropolymer liner with a proximal and a distal cuff, is primarily placed into the jejunum with a delivery catheter. The proximal cuff is anchored at the level of the Z-line of the GE junction and anchored with fullthickness sutures deployed in a circumferential manner. The successor of the ValenTx is a 120 cm long fluorpolymer sleeve which could implement without laparoscopy.

Results: Sandler et al. reported 2018 in sum about 32 obese patients (Mean BMI 42.3Kg/m^2) treated with the successor ValenTx for 12 months. Implantation and removal of the device according to the study concepts was possible in all patients. EWL after one year was 44.8% [20].

Complications: Implantation related AEs were mild (epigastric pain, heartburn or acid reflux, regurgitation, vomiting, dysphagia, and nausea). Longtime AEs were obstructions by knots or kinking. In one patient laparotomy for sleeve explantation was necessary.

6.3 The duodenal mucosal resurfacing (DMR)

DMR potentially mimics some of the mechanisms of action of bariatric surgery in a minimally invasive manner. The DMR procedure is performed using specially designed catheters which are advanced over a guidewire next to the endoscope. It is a single, minimally invasive endoscopic procedure that involves circumferential hydrothermal ablation of the duodenal mucosa resulting in subsequent regeneration of the mucosa. Before ablation, the mucosa is lifted with saline to protect the outer layers of the duodenum. The DMR procedure could be performed under either general anesthesia or deep sedation with propofol.

Results: Van Baar et al. reported 2020 about 37 of 46 patients underwent complete DMR (80%), 36 were finally analyzed; in remaining patients, mainly technical issues were observed [32]. Weight loss was observed in the first 4 weeks, overall was no significant weight loss registered but a significantly decrease of HbA1c and needed anti-diabetic medications. The principle of DMR also allows good glycemic control, but does not lead to significant weight loss [33].

Complications: In the study of Van Baar et al. [32] twenty-four patients had at least one AE (52%) related to DMR. Of these, 81% were mild. One SAE and no unanticipated AEs were reported.

7. Endoscopic bypass

In the context of NOTES development, endoscopically guided gastrojejunal bypass systems have already been developed and successfully performed in the pig model [34]. In the present publications magnets are used, which are applied via the working channel of the scope. These "intelligent" magnets are composed in square or hexagonal form intraluminally. Two such magnets, which act on each other with a force of 600-800 g, cause an anastomosis by reducing the blood supply of the enclosed tissue. This results in a gastro-jejunal [35] or jejuno-ileal [21] anastomosis.

The incisionless magnetic anastomotic system (IMAS; GI Windows, West Bridgewater, MA, USA) is a novel self-assembling magnetic device that allows for side-to-side anastomosis with enteral diversion.

Results: E. Machytka and colleagues [21] performed a prospective, single-arm pilot study, published in 2017. They evaluated the clinical outcomes, safety, and efficacy of IMAS placement and creation of a PJD in a total of 10 patients. At 12 months, patients had an EWL of 40.2%, and a decrease in HbA1c of 1.9% and a decrease in fasting glucose levels of 37% in diabetic patients.

Complications: No adverse events were reported.

8. Others

8.1 SatiSphere

The endoluminal mechanical device is a patent of Endosphere Inc. Columbus, OH, USA for implantation for 3 months. It is implanted endoscopically into the stomach and duodenum through an endoscope under general anesthesia and is composed of a nitinol backbone and spheres made of polyethylenterephtalat with two pigtails at each end. The stent form was made to stay in place by mimicking the anatomy of corresponding parts of the human intestine especially the duodenal C-shape down to the ligament of Treitz.

Results: Sauer et al. [36] reported about 26 treated patients. The study was prematurely terminated.

Complications: Migration of the endoluminal mechanical device was seen in 10/21 patients. Serious adverse events occurred in 10 out of 21 patients in the treatment group.

8.2 Full sense device

This device was introduced 2014 with an internet presentation. The Full Sense Device (Baker, Foote, Kemmeter, Walburn LLC, Grand Rapids, MI) is a temporary, reversible device that is deployed and removed endoscopically. It is a modified fully-covered stent with an esophageal component and a gastric disk component. To stretch the proximal stomach (cardia and fundus) stimulates the vagal nuclei and the vagus nervely. It is designed to induce satiety and fullness in the absence of food by applying pressure on the distal esophagus and gastric cardia.

Results: Only preliminary studies exist. Park and colleagues reported about FSD implantation in 12 pigs [37]. They used fully-covered, partially covered and uncovered stent devices. Luo and colleagues searched for the effects of this system in a rodent model [38].

Complications: There was a high migration rate (11/12) in the porcine model.

9. Endoscopic post-surgical complication management

Relevant early and longtime complications can occur after bariatric surgery. Because the majority of symptomatic patients are endoscopically evaluated, the gastroenterologists must be familiar with post-surgical anatomy and complications, and their endoscopic management.

9.1 Acute complications

9.1.1 Bleeding

Endoluminal hemorrhage after resective procedures in bariatric patients occur with an incidence of up to 5% [39]. Depending on the pathology, endoscopic hemostasis can be achieved by clip (OTSC or TTSC), submucosal injection with fibrin glue or by endoscopic application of hematostyptics.

9.1.2 Anastomotic insufficiency or staple line leaks

The insufficiency of an anastomosis or a staple line leak results in a leakage of enteral fluids into the abdomen. The visceral fat, which is present in pathological amounts, can result in occult peritonitis without typical pain symptoms this conditioned a delay of the detection of the insufficiency. Different endoscopic therapeutic procedures have been established in cases of clinical suspicion of an insufficiency or in cases of proven insufficiencies.

In the case of early detection of insufficiency, re-laparoscopy and, if necessary, overstitching may be appropriate. Often a combination of re-laparoscopy, lavage and drainage for sepsis control and endoscopic therapy is indicated. In hospitals with obesity centers and a 24-hour endoscopy rendezvous procedures with intraoperatively endoscopy could be established. Especially in cases of very small leaks, a reliable identification of the leak can be made [40].

The most frequently performed endoscopic therapy for leakages after bariatric surgery worldwide is the stent therapy [41]. A challenge is the stent fixation in bariatric patients. Stent dislocation is the most common complication of this type of therapy. Special bariatric stents have been developed. The leading brands ECBB HanaroStent® (MI-tech, Seoul, South Korea), MegaStent™ (Taewoong, Seoul, South Korea) and Gastro Seal™ (MI-tech, Seoul, South Korea) are stents 2013 [42]. In addition to the common hemo-clips, the endoscopic sewing machine (EndoStich®, Apollo endosurgery, USA) [43, 44] and a special OTSC (OTSC®Stentfix, Ovesco, Germany) can be used for stent fixation [43].

The endoscopic negative pressure therapy (ENPT) is based on an open-pored element (e.g. a sponge), which is either endoluminally inserted at the stage of the leakage or into the resulting insufficiency cavity (intracavitary). The open-pore element is fixed to a drainage with perforations, which is connected to a vacuum source. The negative pressure acts through the pores on the surrounding tissue and results in a continuous drainage of secretions, cell-detruitus and bacteria, the suction induces tissue proliferation [45]. Due to the good clinical results this therapy is used for numerous leakages of the gastrointestinal and urogenital tract [46, 47]. ENPT is also known under the synonyms E-VAC and EVT. For ENPT as primary endoscopic procedure for leakage, possibly in combination with laparoscopy, three studies are currently available with a cumulative success rate of 90.27% in a total of 31 patients [48–50]. In addition, there are numerous case reports and studies, some of which deal with the combined use of ENPT with stent procedures as first and second line therapy [51].

Closure of leakage after bariatric surgery can be successfully performed with OTSC® as first or second line therapy with good results up to closure rates of 86.3% [52, 53].

The drainage of secretions through an internal drainage by implantation of a double-pigtail-drainage to endoluminal can lead to a successful healing of the insufficiency in up to 78% according to the study results [41].

9.2 Long-time complications

9.2.1 Ulcera

In patients after RYGB, gastrojejunal anastomosis ulceration occurs in up to 16% of cases. Typically, these ulcers occur within 1–6 months postoperatively.

Possible complications of these ulcerations are pain, bleeding and possibly perforations. Endoscopic diagnosis and bleeding therapy can be established as described in "bleeding".

Ulcerations can also occur after gastric banding operations due to the band. In this laparoscopic procedure, an adjustable silicone band is placed around the proximal corpus ventriculi, which causes a deliberate stenosis of the stomach by filling a port appropriately. Erosion of the gastric band can occur in almost 1/3 of the patients [41]. If necessary, the gastric band is then recovered endoscopically [54, 55].

9.2.2 Stenosis

With regard to stenosis after bariatric surgery, the following causes of stenosis should be divided:

- Primary anastomotic stenosis according to RYGB (3–28%) [41, 56],
- Primary stenosis in a sleeve stomach (0.1–3.9%) [57],
- Post-therapeutic stenosis after leakage therapy [41].

Stenosis after bariatric surgery is defined as lumen constriction to less than 10 mm. The therapy consists of an endoscopic controlled balloon dilatation. For the primary stenosis after sleeve gastrectomy (30 mm) achalasia balloons with very good clinical results are used stenosis sleeve.

9.2.3 Weight regain caused by dilated sleeve or gastrojejunal anastomosis

Weight regain after bariatric surgery is a multi-complex problem. While behavioral and genetic mechanisms a dilated gastrojejunal anastomosis (GJA) is a relevante factor of weight recidivism after Roux-en-Y gastric bypass surgery (RYGB).

9.3 TORe with OverStitch™

Endoscopic transoral outlet reduction (TORe) is a therapeutic option for management of weight regain after RYGB. By a full thickness endoscopic suturing device (Overstitch, Apollo Endosurgery, Austin, TX) the reduction of the GJA aperture is possible.

Results: Vargas and colleagues [58] reported in a meta-analysis about 330 patients who underwent TORe procedure. The pooled weight lost at 12 months was 8.4 kg.

Complications: Overall, 14% of patients experienced nausea, 18% had pain and 8% required a repeat EGD. No serious adverse events were reported.

10. OTSC-clip to reduce pouch-outlet and the new BARS device

The OTSC®-clip (Ovesco AG, Tübingen, Germany) is made of super-elastic shape memory alloy (Nitinol) which re-takes its former unbent shape after the clip is released and thus exerts a constant compression on the tissue between the jaws of the clip. In 2020 Ovesco created a new product to reduce pouch-outlet named BARS device (Bariatric Reduction System).

Results: Heylen and colleagues [59] reported about 94 patients who underwent reducing of a post-RYGB pouch-outlet. After one year mean BMI was 27.4 kg/m^2. Di Lorenzo published 2020 results of a clinical trial with BARS device in 6 patients [60]. Authors reported about safely performed procedures with a mean procedure time of 52 min and a mean weight loss of 6 kg at a 3-month FU.

Complications: No SAEs occurred. Some patients complained of a sore throat for 24 h after the intervention. In five patients with post-interventional dysphagia, a gastroscopy had to be performed. Two of patients required endoscopic dilatation.

10.1 StomaphyX device

The transoral StomaphyX device (EndoGastric Solutions) is a minimally invasive technique for revision after RYGB. Procedure seems to be safe and effective.

Results: 2014 Eid et al. [61] published a randomized clinical trial with 45 patients treated with StomaphyX and 25 patients in the sham group. The primary efficacy end point was reduction in pre-RYGB excess weight by 15% or more excess BMI. Patients undergoing StomaphyX treatment experienced significantly greater reduction in weight and BMI. Enrollment was closed prematurely because preliminary results indicated failure to achieve the primary efficacy end point in at least 50% of StomaphyX-treated patients.

Complications: There was one causally related adverse event with StomaphyX that required laparoscopic exploration and repair.

10.2 APC for pouch-outlet reducing

APC is a non-contact technique involving the application of an electrical current to tissues through ionized argon gas (argon plasma). It has also been successfully used in the treatment of the enlargement of the anastomosis after gastric bypass.

Results: Quadros and colleagues [62] published 2020 a randomized controlled trial with APC treatment and sham group. Authors reported about a significant weight decrease in the first months after APC.

Complications: No SAEs were reported.

10.2.1 Choledocholithiasis

The bariatric procedure can be lithogenic due to a hypersecretion of bile and the strong weight loss. A postoperative incidence of cholecystolithiasis in 50% has been described for RYGB. The current guidelines recommends primary cholecystectomy (CHE) in preoperative, symptomatic cholecytolithiasis and, if applicable, in preoperatively known gallstone disease [1]. Simultaneous CHE is not recommended in patients without gallstones. In case of a possibly resulting choledocholithiasis, RYGB is a challenge for the endoscopist. In these cases, laparoscopically assisted ERCP (LA ERCP) or double balloon enteroscopy for the establishment of ERCP (DB ERCP) has become established [41]. Furthermore, there is the possibility to place the duodenoscope laparoscopically assisted via a gastrostomy of the suspended stomach.

11. Conclusion

This overview about the role of endoscopic diagnostic and interventions in obese patients with requiremet of bariatric procedures is certainly not complete and possibly some new and specialized techniques are not listed. Nevertheless we could show the immensely dimension of endoscopy in this field. Endoscopy is an essential part of diagnostics and therapy in the treatment of bariatric patients this applies to the pre- and postoperative phase. As bariatric endoscopy or endoscopic bariatric therapy, a large number of interventions have already been developed, which impress by their minimal invasiveness, low complication rates, manageable costs and good tolerability. Further revolutionary advances in the field of bariatric endoscopy can be expected in the medium term. Interventional endoscopy requires a high level of expertise and a learning curve. It can be expected an increasing number of primary bariatric endoscopic procedures will be performed and bariatric surgery will be relegated to the background due to peri-interventional complications and higher invasiveness.

Abbreviations

ACE	articulating circular endoscopic stapler
AE	adverse event
APC	argon-plasma-coagulation
BMI	body-mass-index
DB	double balloon
DMR	duodenal mucosal resurfacing
EAES	European Association for Endoscopic Surgery
EBT	endoscopic bariatric therapy
EGD	esophago-gastro-duodenoscopy
EGS	endoscopic gastric sleeve
ERCP	endoscopic retrograde cholangio-pancreaticography
ENPT	endoscopic negative-pressure therapy
EVAC	endoscopic vacuum-assisted closure therapy
EVT	endoscopic vacuum-therapy
EWL	excess weight loss
FU	follow-up
GERD	gastro-esophageal reflux disease
IFSO	International Federation for the Surgery of Obesity and Metabolic Disorders
IMAS	incisionless magnetic anastamosis system
IOP	incisionless operating platform
kg	kilogram
LA ERCP	laparoscopic assisted ERCP
LGS	laparoscopic gastric sleeve
m	meter
OTSC	over-the-scope-clip
PEG	percutaneous endoscopic gastrostomy
POSE	primary obesity surgery endoluminal
ROSE	restorative obesity surgery endoluminal
RYGB	Roux-Y-gastric bypass
SAE	severe adverse event
SLL	staple-line-leak
TORe	trans-oral outlet reduction endoscopic
TTSC	through-the-scope-clip
TWL	total weight loss
WHO	World Health Organization

Author details

Dörte Wichmann*, Dietmar Stüker, Ulrich Schweizer, Alfred Königsrainer and Rami Archid
Department of General, Visceral and Transplantation Surgery, University Hospital of Tübingen, Tübingen, Germany

*Address all correspondence to: doerte.wichmann@med.uni-tuebingen.de

References

[1] Di Lorenzo, N., et al., Clinical practice guidelines of the European Association for Endoscopic Surgery (EAES) on bariatric surgery: update 2020 endorsed by IFSO-EC, EASO and ESPCOP. Surg Endosc, 2020. 34(6): p. 2332-2358.

[2] Machytka, E., et al., Adjustable intragastric balloons: a 12-month pilot trial in endoscopic weight loss management. Obes Surg, 2011. 21(10): p. 1499-507.

[3] Usuy, E. and J. Brooks, Response Rates with the Spatz3 Adjustable Balloon. Obes Surg, 2018. 28(5): p. 1271-1276.

[4] Agnihotri, A., et al., *Real-World Safety and Efficacy of Fluid-Filled Dual Intragastric Balloon for Weight Loss.* Clin Gastroenterol Hepatol, 2018. **16**(7): p. 1081-1088 e1.

[5] Force, A.B.E.T., et al., *Endoscopic bariatric therapies.* Gastrointest Endosc, 2015. **81**(5): p. 1073-86.

[6] Marinos, G., et al., *Weight loss and improved quality of life with a nonsurgical endoscopic treatment for obesity: clinical results from a 3- and 6-month study.* Surg Obes Relat Dis, 2014. **10**(5): p. 929-34.

[7] Giardiello, C., et al., *Air-filled vs water-filled intragastric balloon: a prospective randomized study.* Obes Surg, 2012. **22**(12): p. 1916-9.

[8] Lecumberri, E., et al., *Effectiveness and safety of air-filled balloon Heliosphere BAG(R) in 82 consecutive obese patients.* Obes Surg, 2011. **21**(10): p. 1508-12.

[9] Lopez-Nava, G., et al., *The Primary Obesity Surgery Endolumenal (POSE) procedure: one-year patient weight loss and safety outcomes.* Surg Obes Relat Dis, 2015. **11**(4): p. 861-5.

[10] Force, A.B.E.T., et al., *ASGE Bariatric Endoscopy Task Force systematic review and meta-analysis assessing the ASGE PIVI thresholds for adopting endoscopic bariatric therapies.* Gastrointest Endosc, 2015. **82**(3): p. 425-38 e5.

[11] Singh, S., et al., *Safety and efficacy of endoscopic sleeve gastroplasty worldwide for treatment of obesity: a systematic review and meta-analysis.* Surg Obes Relat Dis, 2020. **16**(2): p. 340-351.

[12] Gys, B., et al., *Endoscopic Gastric Plication for Morbid Obesity: a Systematic Review and Meta-analysis of Published Data over Time.* Obes Surg, 2019. **29**(9): p. 3021-3029.

[13] Kumar, N., *Endoscopic therapy for weight loss: Gastroplasty, duodenal sleeves, intragastric balloons, and aspiration.* World J Gastrointest Endosc, 2015. 7(9): p. 847-59.

[14] Fogel, R., et al., *Clinical experience of transoral suturing for an endoluminal vertical gastroplasty: 1-year follow-up in 64 patients.* Gastrointest Endosc, 2008. **68**(1): p. 51-8.

[15] Familiari, P., et al., *Transoral gastroplasty for morbid obesity: a multicenter trial with a 1-year outcome.* Gastrointest Endosc, 2011. **74**(6): p. 1248-58.

[16] Verlaan, T., et al., *Trans-oral Endoscopic Restrictive Implant System: endoscopic treatment of obesity?* Surg Obes Relat Dis, 2016. **12**(9): p. 1711-1718.

[17] Verlaan, T., et al., *Endoscopic gastric volume reduction with a novel articulating plication device is safe and effective in the treatment of obesity (with video).* Gastrointest Endosc, 2015. **81**(2): p. 312-20.

[18] Nystrom, M., et al., *Aspiration Therapy As a Tool to Treat Obesity: 1- to 4-Year Results in a 201-Patient Multi-Center Post-Market European Registry Study.* Obes Surg, 2018. **28**(7): p. 1860-1868.

[19] Betzel, B., et al., *Clinical follow-up on weight loss, glycemic control, and safety aspects of 24 months of duodenal-jejunal bypass liner implantation.* Surg Endosc, 2020. **34**(1): p. 209-215.

[20] Sandler, B.J., et al., *Totally endoscopic implant to effect a gastric bypass: 12-month safety and efficacy outcomes.* Surg Endosc, 2018. **32**(11): p. 4436-4442.

[21] Machytka, E., et al., *Partial jejunal diversion using an incisionless magnetic anastomosis system: 1-year interim results in patients with obesity and diabetes.* Gastrointest Endosc, 2017. **86**(5): p. 904-912.

[22] Ponce, J., et al., *The REDUCE pivotal trial: a prospective, randomized controlled pivotal trial of a dual intragastric balloon for the treatment of obesity.* Surg Obes Relat Dis, 2015. **11**(4): p. 874-81.

[23] Courcoulas, A., et al., *Intragastric balloon as an adjunct to lifestyle intervention: a randomized controlled trial.* Int J Obes (Lond), 2017. **41**(3): p. 427-433.

[24] Force, A.B.E.T., et al., *ASGE position statement on endoscopic bariatric therapies in clinical practice.* Gastrointest Endosc, 2015. **82**(5): p. 767-72.

[25] de Castro, M.L., et al., *Safety and effectiveness of gastric balloons associated with hypocaloric diet for the treatment of obesity.* Rev Esp Enferm Dig, 2013. **105**(9): p. 529-36.

[26] Lopez-Nava, G., et al., *Modified primary obesity surgery endoluminal (POSE-2) procedure for the treatment of obesity.* VideoGIE, 2020. **5**(3): p. 91-93.

[27] Khan, Z., et al., *Efficacy of Endoscopic Interventions for the Management of Obesity: a Meta-analysis to Compare Endoscopic Sleeve Gastroplasty, AspireAssist, and Primary Obesity Surgery Endolumenal.* Obes Surg, 2019. **29**(7): p. 2287-2298.

[28] Sullivan, S., et al., *Randomized sham-controlled trial evaluating efficacy and safety of endoscopic gastric plication for primary obesity: The ESSENTIAL trial.* Obesity (Silver Spring), 2017. **25**(2): p. 294-301.

[29] Huberty, V., et al., *Safety and feasibility of an endoluminal-suturing device for endoscopic gastric reduction (with video).* Gastrointest Endosc, 2017. **85**(4): p. 833-837.

[30] Huberty, V., et al., *Endoscopic gastric reduction with an endoluminal suturing device: a multicenter prospective trial with 1-year follow-up.* Endoscopy, 2018. **50**(12): p. 1156-1162.

[31] Patel, N., et al., *EndoBarrier(R): a Safe and Effective Novel Treatment for Obesity and Type 2 Diabetes?* Obes Surg, 2018. **28**(7): p. 1980-1989.

[32] van Baar, A.C.G., et al., *Endoscopic duodenal mucosal resurfacing for the treatment of type 2 diabetes mellitus: one year results from the first international, open-label, prospective, multicentre study.* Gut, 2020. **69**(2): p. 295-303.

[33] Kumbhari, V., C. Hill, and S. Sullivan, *Bariatric endoscopy: state-of-the-art.* Curr Opin Gastroenterol, 2017. **33**(5): p. 358-365.

[34] Schauer, P., B. Chand, and S. Brethauer, *New applications for endoscopy: the emerging field of endoluminal and transgastric bariatric surgery.* Surg Endosc, 2007. **21**(3): p. 347-56.

[35] Ryou, M., et al., *Smart Self-Assembling MagnetS for ENdoscopy*

(SAMSEN) for transoral endoscopic creation of immediate gastrojejunostomy (with video). Gastrointest Endosc, 2011. **73**(2): p. 353-9.

[36] Sauer, N., et al., *A new endoscopically implantable device (SatiSphere) for treatment of obesity--efficacy, safety, and metabolic effects on glucose, insulin, and GLP-1 levels.* Obes Surg, 2013. **23**(11): p. 1727-33.

[37] Park, J.H., et al., *A Novel Full Sense Device to Treat Obesity in a Porcine Model: Preliminary Results.* Obes Surg, 2019. **29**(5): p. 1521-1527.

[38] Luo, Y., et al., *Intragastric satiety-inducing device reduces food intake and suppresses body weight gain in a rodent model.* Surg Endosc, 2020.

[39] Shikora, S.A. and C.B. Mahoney, *Clinical Benefit of Gastric Staple Line Reinforcement (SLR) in Gastrointestinal Surgery: a Meta-analysis.* Obes Surg, 2015. **25**(7): p. 1133-41.

[40] Wahby, M., et al., *Is routine postoperative gastrografin study needed after laparoscopic sleeve gastrectomy? Experience of 712 cases.* Obes Surg, 2013. **23**(11): p. 1711-7.

[41] Souto-Rodriguez, R. and M.V. Alvarez-Sanchez, *Endoluminal solutions to bariatric surgery complications: A review with a focus on technical aspects and results.* World J Gastrointest Endosc, 2017. **9**(3): p. 105-126.

[42] Puli, S.R., I.S. Spofford, and C.C. Thompson, *Use of self-expandable stents in the treatment of bariatric surgery leaks: a systematic review and meta-analysis.* Gastrointestinal Endoscopy, 2012. **75**(2): p. 287-293.

[43] Chon, S.H., et al., *Efficacy and feasibility of OverStitch suturing of leaks in the upper gastrointestinal tract.* Surg Endosc, 2020. **34**(9): p. 3861-3869.

[44] Bartell, N., et al., *Clinical efficacy of the over-the-scope clip device: A systematic review.* World J Gastroenterol, 2020. **26**(24): p. 3495-3516.

[45] Weidenhagen, R., et al., *Endoscopic vacuum-assisted closure of anastomotic leakage following anterior resection of the rectum: a new method.* Surg Endosc, 2008. **22**(8): p. 1818-25.

[46] Loske, G., *Endoscopic negative pressure therapy of the upper gastrointestinal tract.* Chirurg, 2019. **90**(Suppl 1): p. 1-6.

[47] Loske, G., et al., *Open-pore film drainage (OFD): a new multipurpose tool for endoscopic negative pressure therapy (ENPT).* Endosc Int Open, 2018. **6**(7): p. E865-E871.

[48] Archid, R., et al., *Endoscopic Vacuum Therapy for Staple Line Leaks after Sleeve Gastrectomy.* Obes Surg, 2020. **30**(4): p. 1310-1315.

[49] Leeds, S.G. and J.S. Burdick, *Management of gastric leaks after sleeve gastrectomy with endoluminal vacuum (E-Vac) therapy.* Surg Obes Relat Dis, 2016. **12**(7): p. 1278-1285.

[50] Mencio, M.A., et al., *Use of a novel technique to manage gastrointestinal leaks with endoluminal negative pressure: a single institution experience.* Surgical Endoscopy and Other Interventional Techniques, 2018. **32**(7): p. 3349-3356.

[51] Southwell, T., T.H. Lim, and R. Ogra, *Endoscopic Therapy for Treatment of Staple Line Leaks Post-Laparoscopic Sleeve Gastrectomy (LSG): Experience from a Large Bariatric Surgery Centre in New Zealand.* Obes Surg, 2016. **26**(6): p. 1155-62.

[52] Shoar, S., et al., *Efficacy and Safety of the Over-the-Scope Clip (OTSC) System in the Management of Leak and Fistula After Laparoscopic Sleeve Gastrectomy: a Systematic Review.* Obesity Surgery, 2017. **27**(9): p. 2410-2418.

[53] Keren, D., et al., *Over-the-Scope Clip (OTSC) System for Sleeve Gastrectomy Leaks.* Obesity Surgery, 2015. **25**(8): p. 1358-1363.

[54] Sawicka-Pierko, A., et al., *Gastric band migration to gastrointestinal lumen and possibilities of its surgical treatment.* Advances in Clinical and Experimental Medicine, 2019. **28**(1): p. 103-107.

[55] Himpens, J., et al., *Long-term outcomes of laparoscopic adjustable gastric banding.* Arch Surg, 2011. **146**(7): p. 802-7.

[56] Mathew, A., et al., *Gastrojejunal stricture after gastric bypass and efficacy of endoscopic intervention.* Dig Dis Sci, 2009. **54**(9): p. 1971-8.

[57] Ogra, R. and G.P. Kini, *Evolving Endoscopic Management Options for Symptomatic Stenosis Post-Laparoscopic Sleeve Gastrectomy for Morbid Obesity: Experience at a Large Bariatric Surgery Unit in New Zealand.* Obesity Surgery, 2015. **25**(2): p. 242-248.

[58] Vargas, E.J., et al., *Transoral outlet reduction with full thickness endoscopic suturing for weight regain after gastric bypass: a large multicenter international experience and meta-analysis.* Surg Endosc, 2018. **32**(1): p. 252-259.

[59] Heylen, A.M., et al., *The OTSC(R)-clip in revisional endoscopy against weight gain after bariatric gastric bypass surgery.* Obes Surg, 2011. **21**(10): p. 1629-33.

[60] Di Lorenzo, N., et al., *Bariatric reduction system - BARS: device, technique and first clinical experience.* Minim Invasive Ther Allied Technol, 2020: p. 1-8.

[61] Eid, G.M., et al., *StomaphyX vs a sham procedure for revisional surgery to reduce regained weight in Roux-en-Y gastric bypass patients : a randomized clinical trial.* JAMA Surg, 2014. **149**(4): p. 372-9.

[62] de Quadros, L.G., et al., *Endoscopic Argon Plasma Coagulation vs. Multidisciplinary Evaluation in the Management of Weight Regain After Gastric Bypass Surgery: a Randomized Controlled Trial with SHAM Group.* Obes Surg, 2020. **30**(5): p. 1904-1916.

Chapter 6

Laparoscopic Sleeve Gastrectomy: Outcomes, Safety and Complications

Wahiba Elhag and Walid El Ansari

Abstract

Worldwide, the numbers of laparoscopic sleeve gastrectomy (LSG) performed grown exponentially over the last decade, because of its simplicity, safety profile and excellent outcomes in terms of durable weight loss and improvement of obesity-associated comorbidities. This chapter will provide a comprehensive review on the outcomes of LSG as a metabolic surgery. It appraises LSG's short, mid and long term weight loss outcomes, and compares these outcomes with those of other types of bariatric surgery. Then, a wider range of LSG outcomes are discussed, including a variety of comorbidities, clinical, biochemical and inflammatory parameters, while appraising the positive metabolic effects of LSG. The chapter also outlines the issues pertaining to LSG among a range of special populations such as adolescents, the elderly, renal transplant patients and others. The chapter concludes with a review of the safety and most common complications that may be encountered in the short term and long term, including surgical and nutritional complications, as well as mortality.

Keywords: bariatric surgery, laparoscopic sleeve gastrectomy, technique, perioperative care

1. Introduction

Sleeve gastrectomy (SG) is a restrictive bariatric procedure that was first described as the initial step in biliopancreatic diversion (BPD). Its relative technical ease, effectiveness in weight loss (WL) as a stand-alone procedure, and durability in managing obesity and its comorbid conditions have rendered it the most common bariatric surgery (BS) globally. Below, we discuss the outcomes of LSG.

2. Outcomes

2.1 Anthropometric (weight loss)

WL outcomes after bariatric surgery can be expressed as percentage of excess WL (EWL%) or percentage of excess BMI loss (EBMIL%) [1]. Excess weight is 'ideal body weight subtracted from actual body weight' As for the reporting of the duration of follow up, short-term follow-up is defined as <3 years after intervention, medium-term is ≥3 and <5 years after intervention, and long-term is ≥5 years after intervention [1]. The percentage of excess weight loss (EWL%) varies with the follow-up duration. The average expected EWL% post LSG is 50–60% [2]. A study of 12,129 patients found that the mean EWL% was about 60% at 1 year after surgery, and 65% at 2 years [3]. Midterm (3 years) WL outcomes ranged from 46% to 84.5% [4, 5]. Long term (≥5 years) evidence suggests that although patients regain weight after LSG, they still accomplish a "durable" long-term weight. A review of 277 long-term studies that included 2713 patients revealed a mean 58.4%, 59.5%, 56.6%, 56.4%, and 62.5% EWL% at 5, 6, 7, 8, and 11 years, respectively [6].

When comparing WL outcomes of LSG with other restrictive procedure, LSG was a more effective procedure than laparoscopic adjustable gastric banding (LAGB), contributing to greater WL. For instance, in a review of 33 studies (4109 patients), LSG resulted in significantly higher EWL% compared with LAGB, where mean difference was −16.67% at 12 months, −19.63% at 24 months, and -19.28 at 36 months post surgery [7]. Two Large randomized control trails (RCT) assessed the long-term outcomes of LSG and Roux en Y gastric bypass (RYGB), the Swiss Multicenter Bypass or Sleeve Study (SM-BOSS) [8] and the SLEEVPASS [9]. Both studies reported similar EWL% at 5 years in LSG and RYGB (61.1% vs 68.3%) and (49% and 57%) respectively [8, 9].

2.2 Type 2 Diabetes Mellitus

The improvement in type 2 diabetes mellitus (T2DM) occurs soon after surgery and before considerable WL is achieved, which suggests the existence of weight-independent mechanisms. This is attributed to the changes in the gut hormones, mainly the increase in GLP-1 and the decrease in ghrelin hormone levels post LSG. In the long term, the significant weight loss with LSG leads to improvement in both hepatic and peripheral insulin sensitivity which contributes to T2DM resolution [10]. LSG is associated with significant T2DM improvement. Complete remission rates are 78.3% at 1 year, and 76.2% at 3 years follow up [11]. At 5 years, the remission rate ranged between 60.8% to 71.4% [11, 12].

A body of literature compared the T2DM outcomes of LSG vs conventional medical management [13, 14]. The 5 year outcomes from an RCT (STAMPEDE) that compared intensive medical therapy with BS (LSG or RYGB) found that among 134 individuals, diabetes remission was observed in 5% who received intensive medical therapy alone, compared with 23% who underwent LSG (P = 0.07) [14].

Compared with other restrictive procedures, LSG achieves better T2DM control than LAGB (odds ratio (OR): 0.22, 95% CI: 0.06–0.87, P =0 .03) [7]. LAGB does not cause changes in gut hormones and seem to depend exclusively on restriction for WL and diabetes improvement which might explain the better glycemic control seen after LSG [7]. On the other hand, studies comparing T2DM outcomes between LSG and RYGB reported similar remission rates [8, 9, 15]. A systematic review that included 857 diabetic patients, revealed that T2DM remission rate at 1 year was 63% (LSG) and 74% (RYGB) which were not statistically different [15]. The two RCTs cited previously also confirmed such finding [8, 9].

Several independent factors were identified as predictors of complete T2DM remission, including preoperative HbA1C, EWL%, insulin therapy, age, and oral hypoglycemic medications [11, 16].

2.3 Hypertension and cardiovascular disease

Hypertension has long been associated with obesity. LSG was found to improve hypertension both in the short and the long term [17, 18]. For some hypertensive patients, blood pressure returned to normal on the first day after LSG with a significant reduction observed within 10 days post LSG [17]. The improvement in the blood pressure observed before significant WL suggests other neural and hormonal mechanisms [17]. Over a period of 12 months, hypertension resolved in 87% and improved in 100% of patients [17]. The average number of antihypertensive agents per patient significantly declined from 1.5 to 0.6, and the number of patients requiring >2 antihypertensive agents also fell (baseline 49% vs at 12 months 22%) [17]. On the long-term, hypertension resolved in 62.17% of patients and improved in 35.7% at a mean period of 5.35 years [18]. Moreover, LSG resulted in lower incidence of hypertension on the long term (pre-operative 36.5% vs 14.79% at 5 years), potentially reducing the health system costs [18]. The improvement in hypertension also contributes to a significant 10 year reduction of cardiovascular risk including myocardial infarction and stroke post LSG [19].

2.4 Hyperlipidemia

Hyperlipidemia is a main comorbidity in severe obesity. LSG regulates lipid markers, with considerable reduction in triglyceride, total cholesterol, very low density lipoprotein (VLDL) cholesterol, and low-density lipoprotein (LDL) cholesterol levels, with increase in high-density lipoprotein (HDL) cholesterol level [20, 21]. At 1-year post LSG, remission of hypercholesterolemia and hypertriglyceridemia was attained in 45% and 86% of the patients respectively [20]. Moreover, the improvement observed led to the discontinuation of medication among 43.7% of the patients [20]. On the long term, LSG showed significant improvement in HDL cholesterol and triglyceride compared with preoperative levels [21]. The decreased LDL cholesterol was significant at 1 year and 3 years post surgery, but the effect at 5 years did not reach statistical significance [21]. Overall complete remission of hypercholesteremia at 1, 3 and 5 years was 40.0%, 45.6%, 26.1% respectively [21]. Hypertriglyceridemia remission rate was 72.2%, 66% and 72.2% at 1, 3 and 5 years respectively [21].

2.5 Non-alcoholic fatty liver disease (NAFLD)

NAFLD is liver steatosis in the absence of secondary causes of hepatic fat accumulation such as alcohol abuse. NAFLD can progress to nonalcoholic steatohepatitis (NASH), liver cirrhosis, liver failure, and hepatocellular carcinoma [22]. It is linked to obesity and frequently associated with metabolic syndrome [22]. WL and metabolic improvement post LSG result in a significant improvement in NAFLD. In one study, a liver biopsy was obtained in 134 LSG patients during surgery and 192 days after surgery [23]. There was significant improvement in liver histology following LSG, evident by the improvement in NALFD-Activity-Score (NAS) ($P<0.001$) [23]. NAS is a scoring system developed as a tool to measure changes in NAFLD during therapeutic trials [24]. In the previous study, the percentage of patients with NASH decreased from 18% to 3% [23]. The improvement was greater in severe cases of NAFLD including those with steatohepatitis, bridging fibrosis or cirrhosis. LSG does not only improve the histology and liver function of patients with NAFLD but also reduces the oxidative stress and inflammatory processes involve in the mechanism of NAFLD, where there was significant changes in plasma and liver markers of oxidative stress and inflammation (including chemokine C-C motif ligand 2, paraoxonase-1, galectin-3, and sonic hedgehog) [25]. These data suggest that LSG could be used as therapeutic option to improve NAFLD.

2.6 Obstructive sleep apnea (OSA)

Severe obesity is associated with a high prevalence of moderate-to-severe OSA. A metanalysis showed that at a mean of 24.7 months, LSG resulted in resolution and improvement of sleep apnea in 72% and 51% of patients respectively [26]. One study showed that the apnea hypopnea index significantly decreased from 45.8 to 11.3 events/hour ten months post LSG [27]. The rapid improvement of moderate-to-severe OSA observed post LSG is likely due to the reduced neck circumference. Interestingly, this does not correlate with EWL% which suggests that a weight-independent factors may play a role and hence warrant further research [27].

2.7 Asthma

Obesity is a risk factor for asthma. Many inflammatory markers (e.g. interleukins 5, 6, 13, 17) implicated in the pathogenesis and disease activity of asthma are increased with obesity [28]. WL post LSG results in significantly improved asthma symptoms. A prospective study of 78 subjects compared asthma patients undergoing BS with obese controls. In this study, BS including LSG, resulted in significantly improved small airway function, airway hyperresponsiveness, asthma control and quality of life (QoL) [29]. There was also a decrease in systemic inflammation and bronchial inflammation (mast cell counts) one year after BS [29]. Asthma medication usage was also reduced following LSG [30]. A retrospective analysis of 751 asthmatic patients, including 80 LSG patients, found that the number of prescribed asthma medications among all procedures significantly decreased by 27% at 30 days post-surgery, 37% at 6 months, 44% at 1 year, and 46% at 3 years [30].

2.8 Gastroesophageal reflux disease (GERD)

LSG may improve GERD symptoms as a result of the accelerated gastric emptying and WL. A study of GERD in 65 patients after LSG, including 24-hour pH probe data, suggested that the preexisting reflux improved, and that the de novo reflux rate was low (5.4%) [31]. Appraisal of LSG's effects of on GERD (median follow-up 56 months) using a quality-of-life questionnaire found that GERD-HRQL scores decreased from 7 to 3 [32]. In the same study, GERD-HRQL scores improved in 55 patients, worsened in 21, de novo GERD was observed in 10, and no change in 14 patients [32]. A systematic review (25 studies) reported clinical improvement in 1863 patients at an average of 20 ± 15 months post-LSG; however the review also reported worsening of symptoms in 5953 patients over a period of 29 ± 22 months [33]. However, most research used clinical evaluation, with few studies using endoscopy, 24-hour ambulatory pH, esophageal manometry or contrast studies [33].

2.9 Mental health

Due to the significant association of depression with obesity, it is a common disorder among individuals selected for BS. LSG results in significant improvement in various psychological dimensions. At one year post LSG, depressive symptoms, self-esteem, eating behavior and cognitive restraint showed improving trends [34]. Eating behavior also improves post LSG. In a prospective study of 75 individuals before and 48 months after LSG, the number of patients with binge eating disorder was lower at follow up (decreased from 13% to 2%) [35]. Similarly, the subscales of disinhibition and feelings of hunger both decreased post LSG ($p < 0.001$ for both) [35]. An important outcome post BS is the effect on psychiatric medications, specially depression and anxiety medication. A retrospective study of 50 patients found that at 3- to 6-months post LSG, anxiety symptoms improved in >50% of subjects and most patients were on the same or reduced dosage of medication (62% unchanged, 24% decreased) [36]. Depression symptoms improved in 67%, while 62% of them remained in the same regimen and 26% discontinued their medications

[36]. This suggests that LSG not only results in early improvement in symptoms of depression or anxiety, but also reduces the dosage of psychiatric medications [36].

2.10 Quality of life (QoL)

Morbid obesity together with obesity-related diseases have a negative impact on the QoL. BS, apart from decreasing mortality and morbidity, achieves long-lasting QoL improvement. Significant improvements in physical, psychosocial, and sexual QoL are reported post LSG [37]. QoL and status of general well-being significantly improved 1 to 2 years post LSG [38, 39]. This improvement was also sustained on the long term. For instance, a 10 year follow up study reported significant increase in total QoL before and 10 years after LSG [39]. The global physical health QoL increased from 45.6 ± 20.7 to 62.3 ± 23 at 10 years; the global mental health QoL increased from 49.5 ± 17.7 to 62.2 ± 17.8; and the global total QoL score pre-surgery that was 48.3 ± 20.6 increased to 65.1 ± 21.4 at 10 years [39].

2.11 Biochemical and inflammatory markers

Obesity, especially visceral obesity, is considered as a low-grade inflammatory disease. Serum concentrations of a number of inflammatory markers including C-reactive protein (CRP), tumor necrosis factor-α (TNF-α), and interleukin-6 (IL-6) are elevated in overweight and obese individuals [40]. LSG improves the course of chronic diseases and the state of inflammation associated with obesity. Evidence showed improvements in systemic and urinary inflammatory markers with a significant decrease in interleukin-6 (IL-6), CRP, ferritin, and TNF-α [41]. These changes were also demonstrated in patients with T2DM, where there was significant improvement in inflammatory biomarkers including CRP ($P = 0.003$) and IL-6 at ($P = 0.001$) 6 months post LSG [42]. The reduction in inflammatory factors suggests that LSG may play a role in reducing the risk of T2DM and cardiovascular disease.

2.12 Reproductive systems

2.12.1 Polycystic ovarian syndrome

Polycystic ovarian syndrome (PCOS) is a common endocrine disorder associated with obesity. Women with PCOS have hyperandrogenism and hyperinsulinemia with subsequent insulin resistance and infertility [43]. LSG is effective in treating PCOS, resulting not only in WL, but also significant improvement in the hormonal profile [43, 44]. Significant decrease is observed as early as 3 months post-surgery in luteinizing hormone (LH) levels (7.2 vs. 4.5 mIU/mL), with inversion of LH/FSH ratio ($P = 0.008$), as well as significant decrease in fasting insulin levels (24.4 mIU/mL vs. 9.0 mIU/mL) [44]. LSG also positively augments fertility rates [43, 45]. A cohort of 53 women had a progressive increase of serum anti-Mullerian hormone (marker of ovarian reserve) levels 6 months after LSG [45]. These hormonal changes were also associated with the regulation of the menstrual cycle and resolution of dysmenorrhea [45]. Moreover, 22% percent of PCOS patients became pregnant within 12 months, 69% of which were previously nulliparous [43].

2.12.2 Maternal and perinatal outcomes after LSG

Obese women have increased rates of adverse obstetric outcomes that include gestational diabetes mellitus, gestational hypertension, preeclampsia, cesarean section delivery, and adverse neonatal outcomes including congenital malformations, macrosomia, and stillbirths [46]. WL with LSG has better maternal and perinatal outcomes [47]. A retrospective study comparing women who had undergone LSG with matching controls found that the LSG group had lower rates of gestational DM (3.4% vs 17.6%, P = 0.001), large-for-gestational-age neonates (1.7% vs 19.3%, P = 0.001), and birth weight > 4000 grams (0.8% vs 7.6%, P = 0.02) [47]. Conversely, LSG was associated with higher proportions of small-for-gestational-age (SGA) neonates (14.3% vs 4.2%, P = 0.01) and low-birth-weight neonates (12.6% vs 4.2%, P = 0.03) [47]. Cesarean delivery rates were lower in the LSG group (10.1% vs 20.2%, P = 0.04) [47]. However, LSG patients also had higher risk of iron deficiency anemia requiring treatment with intravenous iron supplementation during pregnancy [47]. This suggests that although LSG improves pregnancy outcomes, however, pregnant women need close monitoring for nutritional deficiencies post LSG.

2.12.3 Male sex hormones

Severe obesity in male patients is accompanied with abnormal sex hormone levels and male hypogonadism. Evidence showed a negative impact of excessive BMI on testosterone levels, sexual function and sperm parameters [48]. LSG is associated with improvement in sexual and reproductive health, and may ameliorate the sex hormone unbalance seen with obesity [49]. The total testosterone levels were significantly increased at 1, 3, 6 months after BS (13.1 ± 7.0, 13.6 ± 5.7, 21.0 ± 19.3 nmol/L, respectively), and estradiol levels significantly decreased at 6 months after surgery (91.4 ± 44.9 pmol/L) [49]. WL with LSG also has favorable effects on semen parameters of patients with pre-existing azoospermia and oligospermia [50]. There was a significant increase in the sperm concentration in men with azoospermia and oligospermia 1 year post LSG (both $P < 0.05$) [50]. Interestingly, the changes in semen and hormones were not affected by the extent of WL experienced by the patients, suggesting an independent mechanism [50].

3. LSG in special populations

3.1 The elderly (>60 years)

Most elderly patients have multiple comorbidities, which are aggravated when severe obesity coexists. Obesity increases their risk of developing cancer, heart disease, diabetes, lower extremity arthritis, sleep apnea, and stroke, with higher mortality risks from cardiovascular disease [51]. LSG is effective for patients older than 65 years resulting in significant WL, comorbidities remission, and improved QoL [52, 53]. LSG for those older than 65 years (median BMI 43 kg/m^2) showed low complications, where only 3.7% had gastric leak with no reported mortality and a median hospital stay of 5 days [52], BMI decreased to 35, 32.9 and 30.7 kg/m^2 at 6, 12 and 24 months after LSG and the mean EWL was 76.3% at 2 years [52]. Moreover, T2DM, hypertension, dyslipidemia, OSA, and arthralgia showed significant remission at 1 and 2 years following LSG [52]. As for QoL, there was also significant improvement in the scales that represent physical health, mental health (social function), general health perception and vitality scores [52].

3.2 Adolescents

Severe obesity in adolescents is associated with multiple comorbidities such as T2DM, hypertension, sleep apnea, fatty liver disease, decreased QoL and cardiovascular mortality in adulthood [54]. LSG has become the most used operation among adolescents with severe obesity mainly because of comparable WL outcomes and morbidities resolution to RYGB [55]. Moreover, LSG carries lower risk of surgical and nutritional complications [55, 56]. Indications for BS in adolescents largely mirrors the recommendations for adults [54]. There are no data to suggest that a youth's puberty status or linear growth is adversely affected by BS. A study showed improved linear growth in children after LSG compared with matched controls [57]. LSG results is significant WL, with EWL% at one year ranging from 49% to 81% [56, 58], and with durable long term WL (78%) (5 years) [58]. In terms of comorbidities, surgical treatment of adolescents with severe obesity and T2DM resulted in superior glycemic control than medical treatment. Across two different studies, the Teen-Longitudinal Assessment of BS (Teen-LABS) and the Treatment Options of Type 2 Diabetes in Adolescents and Youth (TODAY) study, a comparison of the glycemic control data showed that at 2 years, the mean hemoglobin A1c concentration decreased from 6.8% to 5.5% in Teen-LABS and increased from 6.4% to 7.8 in the TODAY study [55]. At 5 years post LSG, the remission rate of insulin resistance and T2DM was 100% and 87% respectively [58]. LSG also has a favorable outcome in terms of improvement of nonalcoholic steatohepatitis (NASH) [59]. Among adolescents who underwent LSG, NASH reverted completely in all patients and hepatic fibrosis stage 2 disappeared in 90% of the patients [59]. Moreover, LSG resulted in marked and sustained improvements in HRQoL, weight-related QoL and body image satisfaction [55, 60].

3.3 Low BMI

BS promotes marked and durable resolution of the clinical manifestations of diabetes in morbidly obese patients with T2DM. However, among Asians, the risks associated with T2DM and cardiovascular disease occur at a lower BMI than in Whites [61]. Patients with BMI < 35 kg/m^2 who have uncontrolled and life-threatening comorbidities do not meet the traditional criteria for obesity surgery. A surgical approach may be appropriate as an alternative for inadequately controlled T2DM in suitable surgical candidates with mild to moderate obesity (BMI 30–35 kg/m^2) [62].

3.3.1 Class I obesity (< 30 BMI)

For patients with BMI < 30 kg/m^2, a meta-analysis (12 studies, including 697 Asians) found that at 12 months postoperatively, BMI and waist circumference were reduced by 2.88 kg/m^2 and 12.92 cm, respectively [61]. There was a significant improvement in glycemic control, lipid profiles, and β-cell function in the short and medium terms (6–24 months) [61]. A study of 25 Asians with T2DM and BMI of 23.23 to 29.97 kg/m^2 showed that the complete remission rates at 3, 6, and 12 months postoperatively for T2DM were 40%, 60%, 68% respectively, hypertension (22.2%, 50%, 75% respectively), hypertriglyceridemia (66.7%, 66.7%, 100% respectively), and hypercholesterolemia (41.7%, 60%, 100% respectively) [63].

3.3.2 Class II obesity (<35 BMI)

In a randomized controlled trial where 34% of the patients had BMI < 35 kg/m^2, WL and diabetes remission were greater post LSG than after conventional treatment, and were comparable to RYGB [64]. Midterm follow-up (3 years) of 252 patients with BMI < 35 showed %EWL of 75.8% [65]. Insulin resistance remitted in 89.4%, dyslipidemia in 52%, NAFLD in 84.6%, hypertension in 75% and GERD in 65% [65]. T2DM showed 60% complete remission and 40% improvement [65].

The morbidity rate was 2.4%, two patients required reoperations, and no leaks or mortality were reported [65]. This suggests that LSG in patients with BMI < 35 kg/m^2 is safe and effective, and BMI should not be the only indicator to consider BS. Further studies with longer follow-ups are required.

3.4 Renal transplant patients

Morbid obesity is a barrier to kidney transplantation due to inferior outcomes, higher rates of new-onset diabetes after transplantation, delayed graft function, and graft failure [66]. LSG improves renal transplant candidacy and post transplant outcomes in morbidly obese patients [67, 68]. Kidney recipients who underwent LSG were compared with similar BMI recipients who did not undergo LSG [67]. In this study, the BMI decreased from 41.5 to 32.3 kg/m^2, with no complications, readmissions, or mortality following LSG [67]. After transplantation, one patient experienced delayed graft function and no other patients had new-onset diabetes [67]. Moreover, allograft survival and patient survival at 1-year post transplantation were 100% [67]. Compared with non-LSG patients, post-LSG recipients had significantly lower delayed graft function rates and renal dysfunction-related readmissions [67]. Longer duration studies showed that LSG in patients with obesity and end-stage kidney disease was associated with lower all-cause mortality at 5 years compared with usual care (cumulative incidence 25.6% vs 39.8%; hazard ratio 0.69, 95% CI, 0.60–0.78), which is likely driven by the lower mortality from cardiovascular disease [68]. Moreover, LSG was associated with an increased rate of kidney transplant at 5 years (cumulative incidence 33.0% vs 20.4%; hazard ratio 1.82; 95% CI, 1.58–2.09) [68].

3.5 Inflammatory bowel disease (IBD)

Historically, IBD patients were unlikely to be overweight or obese due to the malabsorption and catabolic disease state; however, the increasing rates of obesity along with enhanced therapeutics have now resulted in higher incidence of obese patients. The prevalence of obesity and severe obesity among IBD patients is about 20–30% and 2–5%, respectively [69]. LSG is safer compared with RYGB for IBD patients as immunosuppressant drugs might place IBD patients at higher risk of surgical complications. The underlying nutritional deficiencies in IBD patients may also increase susceptibility to micronutrient deficiencies after BS. Moreover, IBD could increase the conversion rate of laparoscopic to open surgeries [70]. Despite these concerns, studies have found that LSG has favorable outcomes in patients with IBD. For example, one study showed that among patients with Crohn's disease (CD) or ulcerative colitis (UC) who underwent RYGB (n= 19) and LSG (n= 35), both operations led to significant WL at 1 year [71]. Additionally, a sizable proportion of patients experienced improvements in IBD after RYGB and LSG [71]. There were no significant differences in the proportion of patients with UC who had improved (27% vs 8%), unchanged (64% vs 92%), or worse (9% vs 0%) IBD medication requirements, respectively [71]. Similar analysis among patients with CD showed no significant differences in the proportion of patients who had improved (37.5% vs 44%) or unchanged (25% vs 52%) IBD-medication requirements after RYGB and LSG, respectively. However, there was a significant difference in the proportion of patients who had worsened CD after RYGB compared with LSG (37.5% vs 4%, $p = 0.016$) [71]. In terms of complications, a metanalysis (10 studies) favored LSG over RYGB for early (<30 days) complications (LSG 14.9% vs RYGB 28.9%) and late (>30 days) complications (LSG 15.0% vs RYGB 26.8%) [70].

4. Safety and complications

The rate of major complications after LSG is 0–6% [72, 73]. Early complications include leak, bleeding, symptomatic stenosis, deep vien thrombosis/pulmonary embolism (DVT/PE), risk of portomesenteric venous thrombosis, and dehydration. Late complications include stricture, weight regain, and malnutrition.

4.1 30-day morbidity and mortality

Mortality after LSG is currently low. A large study that included 134,142 patients where 69% of patients underwent LSG and 31% had RYGB found that the mortality and morbidity rates were significantly lower in LSG compared with RYGB (0.1% vs 0.2%; 5.8% vs 11.7%, respectively). The most important predictors of morbidity and mortality outcomes were BMI, albumin, and age [74].

4.2 Leak

Leak rates range from 0.5–7.0%, though most recent reported leak rate is about 1%, reflecting improvements with time and experience in the LSG technique [73, 75]. Gastric leak can result from mechanical forces that stress the staple line or ischemia. About 75–85% of LSG leaks occur at the proximal third of the greater curvature staple line, as opposed to the distal or antral staple line, and usually occur at postoperative day 5 or later [75]. Clinically, post-LSG leak presents with left upper quadrant pain, tachycardia, fever, or leukocytosis. Upper gastrointestinal contrast studies have low sensitivity (0–25%) but high specificity (90–95%) [72]. Due to its greater sensitivity, computerized tomography (CT) scan with oral and intravenous contrast is now used for diagnosis of a leak in clinically stable patients with suggestive signs or symptoms [72]. For acute postoperative leak, patients who are not stable enough for CT should be returned to the operating room for diagnostic laparoscopy. In acute leak, the objective is adequate drainage to prevent or mitigate abdominal sepsis. Treatment includes adequate drainage, nutritional support, and antibiotics. In most cases, resolution of the leak is a matter of time, sometimes taking several months [76]. Endoscopic treatments are increasingly utilized with variable success rates in an effort to avoid surgical interventions [77].

4.3 Stenosis

Stenosis can result from the surgical technique or ischemia with subsequent stricture development. Clinically, significant stenosis occurs in 0.5–3.5% of cases, most often in a short segment located at mid-body, near the incisura [78]. Diagnosis is made by upper gastrointestinal contrast studies. Initial management is endoscopic balloon dilatation, probably requiring 2–4 dilation sessions, with 95–100% long-term success rates [79]. However, there is a 2–5% risk of perforation associated with dilation [72]. For cases where endoscopic dilation fails, the options include endoscopic stenting or conversion to RYGB [80].

4.4 Hemorrhage

Postoperative hemorrhage is rare after LSG and less common than with RYGB. Bleeding usually occurs at the staple line and is extraluminal in about half of the cases. CT scan confirms the diagnosis, and emergency surgical intervention is required for clinically significant active hemorrhage. For intraluminal bleeding, endoscopic interventions, including epinephrine injection, heater probe, and clipping, are effective [72].

4.5 GERD

Significant GERD is considered a contraindication for LSG. Some studies show an increased prevalence of GERD in patients after LSG. This is likely due to hypotensive lower esophageal sphincter, disruption of the angle of His, reduced gastric compliance with higher intragastric pressure, and decreased gastric emptying. Late dilatation of the sleeve, and occurrence of hiatal hernia could also play a role in the worsening of GERD [81]. It is not recommended to empirically start antacid medication for prophylaxis after LSG [82]. However, for patients who develop reflux after LSG, treatment options are proton-pump inhibitors or conversion to RYGB [83].

4.6 Portomesenteric venous thrombosis

Portomesenteric venous thrombosis is a rare complication of LSG thought to be secondary to regional postsurgical inflammation, change in venous outflow, and dehydration predisposing to clot formation [72]. Patients may present 1–2 weeks after surgery with vague abdominal pain, severe nausea and vomiting, fever and diffuse abdominal tenderness. Diagnosis is confirmed with CT scan. Treatment consists of anticoagulation, fluid resuscitation, and bowel rest. Thrombolytics may be indicated depending on severity of symptoms. There are no established guidelines for the duration of anticoagulation therapy, but patients are usually treated for 3–6 months. Surgical treatment is reserved for patients with evidence of infarcted bowel [84].

4.7 Nutritional deficiencies

Although LSG is viewed as a restrictive procedure, some degree of malabsorption is also expected. After recovering from surgery, patients are at risk of macronutrient deficiencies in the long term due to reduced dietary intake, decreased gastric secretion of hydrochloric acid and intrinsic factor, and poor food choices. The most common micronutrient deficiencies are of vitamins B12 and D, iron, and calcium [85]. Other micronutrient deficiencies that can lead to severe complications include thiamine, folate, and fat-soluble vitamins [85]. Daily micronutrient supplements are necessary, including multivitamin concentrate (with iron, copper, and zinc), calcium citrate with vitamin D, vitamin B12, and elemental iron [82]. However, multivitamins or nutritional supplements are typically not initiated in the immediate postoperative period [82]. It is necessary to clinically monitor the bariatric patient during the first five years. Some evidence suggests that patients experienced fewer nutrient deficiencies after LSG than after RYGB [86].

4.8 Mortality

Mortality after LSG is currently low according to data from the American College of Surgeons - BS Center Network (includes 28616 patients in 25 hospitals in the USA), where the 30-day mortality was 0.11% and the 1 year mortality was 0.21% [87].

5. Conclusion

Since its evolution from the initial step of a staged procedure to a stand-alone procedure, LSG has emerged as the most commonly performed bariatric operation worldwide. This is due to its technical ease, coupled with decreased surgical complications in comparison with other more complex surgical procedures. It has proven to be safe and effective in achieving weight loss and addressing the metabolic derangements associated with obesity. In addition, long term outcomes have demonstrated that the durability of LSG is comparable with that of other bariatric procedures.

Conflict of interest

None.

Author details

Wahiba Elhag[1] and Walid El Ansari[2,3,4*]

1 Department of Bariatric Surgery/Bariatric Medicine, Hamad General Hospital, Doha, Qatar

2 Department of Surgery, Hamad General Hospital, Doha, Qatar

3 College of Medicine, Qatar University, Doha, Qatar

4 Schools of Health and Education, University of Skovde, Skövde, Sweden

*Address all correspondence to: welansari9@gmail.com

References

[1] Brethauer SA, Kim J, el Chaar M, et al. Standardized outcomes reporting in metabolic and bariatric surgery. Surg Obes Relat Dis. 2015;**11**:489-506

[2] Mechanick JI, Apovian C, Brethauer S, et al. Clinical practice guidelines for the perioperative nutrition, metabolic, and nonsurgical support of patients undergoing bariatric procedures - 2019 update: cosponsored by American Association of Clinical Endocrinologists/ American College of Endocrinology, The Obesity Society, American Society for Metabolic & Bariatric Surgery, Obesity Medicine Association, and American Society of Anesthesiologists. Surg Obes Relat Dis. 2020;**16**:175-247

[3] Fischer L, Hildebrandt C, Bruckner T, et al. Excessive weight loss after sleeve gastrectomy: a systematic review. Obes Surg. 2012;**22**:721-731

[4] Lemanu DP, Singh PP, Rahman H, Hill AG, Babor R, MacCormick AD. Five-year results after laparoscopic sleeve gastrectomy: a prospective study. Surg Obes Relat Dis. 2015;**11**:518-524

[5] Boza C, Salinas J, Salgado N, Pérez G, Raddatz A, Funke R, et al. Laparoscopic sleeve gastrectomy as a stand-alone procedure for morbid obesity: report of 1,000 cases and 3-year follow-up. Obes Surg. 2012;**22**:866-871

[6] Juodeikis Ž, Brimas G. Long-term results after sleeve gastrectomy: A systematic review. Surg Obes Relat Dis. 2017;**13**:693-699

[7] Li L, Yu H, Liang J, Guo Y, Peng S, Luo Y, et al. Meta-analysis of the effectiveness of laparoscopic adjustable gastric banding versus laparoscopic sleeve gastrectomy for obesity. Medicine (Baltimore). 2019;**98**:e14735

[8] Peterli R, Wölnerhanssen BK, Peters T, et al. Effect of Laparoscopic Sleeve Gastrectomy vs Laparoscopic Roux-en-Y Gastric Bypass on Weight Loss in Patients With Morbid Obesity: The SM-BOSS Randomized Clinical Trial. JAMA. 2018;**319**:255-265

[9] Salminen P, Helmiö M, Ovaska J, et al. Effect of Laparoscopic Sleeve Gastrectomy vs Laparoscopic Roux-en-Y Gastric Bypass on Weight Loss at 5 Years Among Patients With Morbid Obesity. JAMA. 2018;**319**:241-254

[10] Jiménez A, Casamitjana R, Flores L, Delgado S, Lacy A, Vidal J. GLP-1 and the long-term outcome of type 2 diabetes mellitus after Roux-en-Y gastric bypass surgery in morbidly obese subjects. Ann Surg. 2013;**257**:894-899

[11] Viscido G, Gorodner V, Signorini FJ, et al. Obese Patients with Type 2 Diabetes: Outcomes After Laparoscopic Sleeve Gastrectomy. J Laparoendosc Adv Surg Tech A. 2019;**29**:655-662

[12] Switzer NJ, Prasad S, Debru E, Church N, Mitchell P, Gill RS. Sleeve Gastrectomy and Type 2 Diabetes Mellitus: a Systematic Review of Long-Term Outcomes. Obes Surg. 2016;**26**:1616-1621

[13] Gu J, Vergis A. Diabetes improvement and bariatric surgery—review of laparoscopic Roux-en-Y gastric bypass vs. laparoscopic vertical sleeve gastrectomy. Ann Transl Med [Internet]. 2020 [cited 2020 Aug 12];8.

[14] Schauer PR, Bhatt DL, Kirwan JP, et al. Bariatric Surgery versus Intensive Medical Therapy for Diabetes - 5-Year Outcomes. N Engl J Med. 2017;**376**:641-651

[15] Cho J-M, Kim HJ, Lo Menzo E, Park S, Szomstein S, Rosenthal RJ. Effect of sleeve gastrectomy on type 2

diabetes as an alternative treatment modality to Roux-en-Y gastric bypass: systemic review and meta-analysis. Surg Obes Relat Dis. 2015;**11**:1273-1280

[16] Elgenaied I, El Ansari W, Elsherif MA, Abdulrazzaq S, Qabbani AS, Elhag W. Factors associated with complete and partial remission, improvement, or unchanged diabetes status of obese adults 1 year after sleeve gastrectomy. Surg Obes Relat Dis. 2020; May 27:S1550-7289(20)30271-9. doi: 10.1016/j.soard.2020.05.013. Online ahead of print.

[17] Yin X, Qian J, Wang Y, et al. Short-term outcome and early effect on blood pressure of laparoscopic sleeve gastrectomy in morbidly obese patients. Clin Exp Hypertens. 2019;**41**:622-626

[18] Graham C, Switzer N, Reso A, et al. Sleeve gastrectomy and hypertension: a systematic review of long-term outcomes. Surg Endosc. 2019;**33**:3001-3007

[19] Blanco DG, Funes DR, Giambartolomei G, Lo Menzo E, Szomstein S, Rosenthal RJ. Laparoscopic sleeve gastrectomy versus Roux-en Y gastric bypass in cardiovascular risk reduction: A match control study. Surg Obes Relat Dis. 2019;**15**:14-20

[20] Vigilante A, Signorini F, Marani M, et al. Impact on Dyslipidemia After Laparoscopic Sleeve Gastrectomy. Obes Surg. 2018;**28**:3111-3115

[21] Golomb I, Ben David M, Glass A, Kolitz T, Keidar A. Long-term Metabolic Effects of Laparoscopic Sleeve Gastrectomy. JAMA Surg. 2015;**150**:1051-1057

[22] Marchisello S, Di Pino A, Scicali R, et al. Pathophysiological, Molecular and Therapeutic Issues of Nonalcoholic Fatty Liver Disease: An Overview. Int J Mol Sci [Internet]. 2019 [cited 2020 Aug 13];20.

[23] von Schönfels W, Beckmann JH, Ahrens M, et al. Histologic improvement of NAFLD in patients with obesity after bariatric surgery based on standardized NAS (NAFLD activity score). Surg Obes Relat Dis. 2018;**14**:1607-1616

[24] Brunt EM, Kleiner DE, Wilson LA, Belt P, Neuschwander-Tetri BA. The NAS and The Histopathologic Diagnosis in NAFLD: Distinct Clinicopathologic Meanings. Hepatology. 2011;**53**:810-820

[25] Cabré N, Luciano-Mateo F, Fernández-Arroyo S, et al. Laparoscopic sleeve gastrectomy reverses non-alcoholic fatty liver disease modulating oxidative stress and inflammation. Metab Clin Exp. 2019;**99**:81-89

[26] Sarkhosh K, Switzer NJ, El-Hadi M, Birch DW, Shi X, Karmali S. The impact of bariatric surgery on obstructive sleep apnea: a systematic review. Obes Surg. 2013;**23**:414-423

[27] Timmerman M, Basille D, Basille-Fantinato A, et al. Short-Term Assessment of Obstructive Sleep Apnea Syndrome Remission Rate after Sleeve Gastrectomy: a Cohort Study. Obes Surg. 2019;**29**:3690-3697

[28] Mohan A, Grace J, Wang BR, Lugogo N. The Effects of Obesity in Asthma. Curr Allergy Asthma Rep. 2019;**19**:49

[29] van Huisstede A, Rudolphus A, Castro Cabezas M, et al. Effect of bariatric surgery on asthma control, lung function and bronchial and systemic inflammation in morbidly obese subjects with asthma. Thorax. 2015;**70**:659-667

[30] Guerron AD, Ortega CB, Lee H-J, Davalos G, Ingram J, Portenier D. Asthma medication usage is significantly reduced following bariatric surgery. Surg Endosc. 2019;**33**:1967-1975

[31] Rebecchi F, Allaix ME, Giaccone C, Ugliono E, Scozzari G, Morino M. Gastroesophageal reflux disease and laparoscopic sleeve gastrectomy: a physiopathologic evaluation. Ann Surg. 2014;**260**:909-914 discussion 914-915

[32] Balla A, Quaresima S, Palmieri L, et al. Effects of Laparoscopic Sleeve Gastrectomy on Quality of Life Related to Gastroesophageal Reflux Disease. J Laparoendosc Adv Surg Tech A. 2019;**29**:1532-1538

[33] Stenard F, Iannelli A. Laparoscopic sleeve gastrectomy and gastroesophageal reflux. World J Gastroenterol. 2015;**21**:10348-10357

[34] Çalışır S, Çalışır A, Arslan M, İnanlı İ, Çalışkan AM, Eren İ. Assessment of depressive symptoms, self-esteem, and eating psychopathology after laparoscopic sleeve gastrectomy: 1-year follow-up and comparison with healthy controls. Eat Weight Disord. 2019; 2019;10.1007/s40519-019-00785-7. doi:10.1007/s40519-019-00785-7. Online ahead of print.

[35] Mack I, Ölschläger S, Sauer H, et al. Does Laparoscopic Sleeve Gastrectomy Improve Depression, Stress and Eating Behaviour? A 4-Year Follow-up Study. Obes Surg. 2016;**26**:2967-2973

[36] Monte SV, Russo KM, Mustafa E, Caruana JA. Impact of Sleeve Gastrectomy on Psychiatric Medication Use and Symptoms. J Obes [Internet]. 2018 [cited 2020 Aug 1];2018.

[37] Brunault P, Frammery J, Couet C, et al. Predictors of changes in physical, psychosocial, sexual quality of life, and comfort with food after obesity surgery: a 12-month follow-up study. Qual Life Res. 2015;**24**:493-501

[38] Charalampakis V, Bertsias G, Lamprou V, de Bree E, Romanos J, Melissas J. Quality of life before and after laparoscopic sleeve gastrectomy. A prospective cohort study. Surg Obes Relat Dis. 2015;**11**:70-76

[39] Major P, Matłok M, Pędziwiatr M, et al. Quality of Life After Bariatric Surgery. Obes Surg. 2015;**25**:1703-1710

[40] Faam B, Zarkesh M, Daneshpour MS, Azizi F, Hedayati M. The association between inflammatory markers and obesity-related factors in Tehranian adults: Tehran lipid and glucose study. Iran J Basic Med Sci. 2014;**17**:577-582

[41] Gumbau V, Bruna M, Canelles E, et al. A prospective study on inflammatory parameters in obese patients after sleeve gastrectomy. Obes Surg. 2014;**24**:903-908

[42] Mallipedhi A, Prior SL, Barry JD, Caplin S, Baxter JN, Stephens JW. Changes in inflammatory markers after sleeve gastrectomy in patients with impaired glucose homeostasis and type 2 diabetes. Surg Obes Relat Dis. 2014;**10**:1123-1128

[43] Dilday J, Derickson M, Kuckelman J, et al. Sleeve Gastrectomy for Obesity in Polycystic Ovarian Syndrome: a Pilot Study Evaluating Weight Loss and Fertility Outcomes. Obes Surg. 2019;**29**:93-98

[44] Machado Júnior AS, Ribeiro CBL, Santa-Cruz F, et al. The Effect of Sleeve Gastrectomy on the Hormonal Profile of Patients with Polycystic Ovary Syndrome. Obes Surg. 2019;**29**:2415-2419

[45] Pilone V, Tramontano S, Renzulli M, et al. Evaluation of anti-Müller hormone AMH levels in obese women after sleeve gastrectomy. Gynecol Endocrinol. 2019;**35**:548-551

[46] Schummers L, Hutcheon JA, Bodnar LM, Lieberman E, Himes KP. Risk of adverse pregnancy outcomes by prepregnancy body mass index: a population-based study to inform

prepregnancy weight loss counseling. Obstet Gynecol. 2015;**125**:133-143

[47] Rottenstreich A, Elchalal U, Kleinstern G, Beglaibter N, Khalaileh A, Elazary R. Maternal and Perinatal Outcomes After Laparoscopic Sleeve Gastrectomy. Obstet Gynecol. 2018;**131**:451-456

[48] Mihalca R, Fica S. The impact of obesity on the male reproductive axis. J Med Life. 2014;**7**:296-300

[49] Zhu C, Zhang Y, Wang X, et al. Effect of laparoscopic sleeve gastrectomy on sex hormone in male severe obesity. Zhonghua Wei Chang Wai Ke Za Zhi. 2017;**20**:405-410

[50] El Bardisi H, Majzoub A, Arafa M, et al. Effect of bariatric surgery on semen parameters and sex hormone concentrations: a prospective study. Reprod Biomed Online. 2016;**33**:606-611

[51] Zamboni M, Mazzali G, Zoico E, et al. Health consequences of obesity in the elderly: a review of four unresolved questions. Int J Obes (Lond). 2005;**29**:1011-29.

[52] Lainas P, Dammaro C, Gaillard M, Donatelli G, Tranchart H, Dagher I. Safety and short-term outcomes of laparoscopic sleeve gastrectomy for patients over 65 years old with severe obesity. Surg Obes Relat Dis. 2018;**14**:952-959

[53] Dowgiałło-Wnukiewicz N, Janik MR, Lech P, et al. Outcomes of sleeve gastrectomy in patients older than 60 years: a multicenter matched case-control study. Wideochir Inne Tech Maloinwazyjne. 2020;**15**:123-128

[54] Pratt JSA, Browne A, Browne NT, et al. ASMBS pediatric metabolic and bariatric surgery guidelines, 2018. Surg Obes Relat Dis. 2018;**14**:882-901

[55] Inge TH, Courcoulas AP, Jenkins TM, et al. Weight Loss and Health Status 3 Years after Bariatric Surgery in Adolescents. N Engl J Med. 2016;**374**:113-123

[56] Elhag W, El Ansari W, Abdulrazzaq S, Abdullah A, Elsherif M, Elgenaied I. Evolution of 29 Anthropometric, Nutritional, and Cardiometabolic Parameters Among Morbidly Obese Adolescents 2 Years Post Sleeve Gastrectomy. Obes Surg. 2018;**28**:474-482

[57] Alqahtani A, Elahmedi M, Qahtani ARA. Laparoscopic Sleeve Gastrectomy in Children Younger Than 14 Years: Refuting the Concerns. Ann Surg. 2016;**263**:312-319

[58] Khidir N, El-Matbouly MA, Sargsyan D, Al-Kuwari M, Bashah M, Gagner M. Five-year Outcomes of Laparoscopic Sleeve Gastrectomy: a Comparison Between Adults and Adolescents. Obes Surg. 2018;**28**:2040-2045

[59] Manco M, Mosca A, De Peppo F, et al. The Benefit of Sleeve Gastrectomy in Obese Adolescents on Nonalcoholic Steatohepatitis and Hepatic Fibrosis. J Pediatr. 2017;**180**:31-37.e2.

[60] El-Matbouly MA, Khidir N, Touny HA, El Ansari W, Al-Kuwari M, Bashah M. A 5-Year Follow-Up Study of Laparoscopic Sleeve Gastrectomy Among Morbidly Obese Adolescents: Does It Improve Body Image and Prevent and Treat Diabetes? Obes Surg. 2018;**28**:513-519

[61] Ji G, Li P, Li W, et al. The Effect of Bariatric Surgery on Asian Patients with Type 2 Diabetes Mellitus and Body Mass Index < 30 kg/m2: a Systematic Review and Meta-analysis. Obes Surg. 2019;**29**:2492-2502

[62] Rubino F, Nathan DM, Eckel RH, et al. Metabolic Surgery in the Treatment Algorithm for Type 2 Diabetes: A Joint Statement by

International Diabetes Organizations. Diabetes Care. 2016;**39**:861-877

[63] Wang L, Wang J, Jiang T. Effect of Laparoscopic Sleeve Gastrectomy on Type 2 Diabetes Mellitus in Patients with Body Mass Index less than 30 kg/m2. Obes Surg. 2019;**29**:835-842

[64] Schauer PR, Kashyap SR, Wolski K, et al. Bariatric surgery versus intensive medical therapy in obese patients with diabetes. N Engl J Med. 2012;**366**:1567-1576

[65] Berry MA, Urrutia L, Lamoza P, et al. Sleeve Gastrectomy Outcomes in Patients with BMI Between 30 and 35-3 Years of Follow-Up. Obes Surg. 2018;**28**:649-655

[66] Sood A, Hakim DN, Hakim NS. Consequences of Recipient Obesity on Postoperative Outcomes in a Renal Transplant: A Systematic Review and Meta-Analysis. Exp Clin Transplant. 2016;**14**:121-128

[67] Kim Y, Jung AD, Dhar VK, et al. Laparoscopic sleeve gastrectomy improves renal transplant candidacy and posttransplant outcomes in morbidly obese patients. Am J Transplant. 2018;**18**:410-416

[68] Sheetz KH, Gerhardinger L, Dimick JB, Waits SA. Bariatric Surgery and Long-term Survival in Patients With Obesity and End-stage Kidney Disease. JAMA Surg. 2020;

[69] Steed H, Walsh S, Reynolds N. A brief report of the epidemiology of obesity in the inflammatory bowel disease population of Tayside. Scotland. Obes Facts. 2009;**2**:**370**-372

[70] Garg R, Mohan BP, Ponnada S, Singh A, Aminian A, Regueiro M, et al. Safety and Efficacy of Bariatric Surgery in Inflammatory Bowel Disease Patients: a Systematic Review and Meta-analysis. Obes Surg. 2020; 10.1007/s11695-020-04729-4. doi:10.1007/s11695-020-04729-4. Online ahead of print.

[71] Heshmati K, Lo T, Tavakkoli A, Sheu E. Short-Term Outcomes of Inflammatory Bowel Disease after Roux-en-Y Gastric Bypass vs Sleeve Gastrectomy. J Am Coll Surg. 2019;**228**:893-901.e1

[72] Chung AY, Thompson R, Overby DW, Duke MC, Farrell TM. Sleeve Gastrectomy: Surgical Tips. J Laparoendosc Adv Surg Tech A. 2018;**28**:930-937

[73] Stroh C, Köckerling F, Volker L, et al. Results of More Than 11,800 Sleeve Gastrectomies: Data Analysis of the German Bariatric Surgery Registry. Ann Surg. 2016;**263**:949-955

[74] Kumar SB, Hamilton BC, Wood SG, Rogers SJ, Carter JT, Lin MY. Is laparoscopic sleeve gastrectomy safer than laparoscopic gastric bypass? a comparison of 30-day complications using the MBSAQIP data registry. Surg Obes Relat Dis. 2018;**14**:264-269

[75] Kim J, Azagury D, Eisenberg D, DeMaria E, Campos GM. American Society for Metabolic and Bariatric Surgery Clinical Issues Committee. ASMBS position statement on prevention, detection, and treatment of gastrointestinal leak after gastric bypass and sleeve gastrectomy, including the roles of imaging, surgical exploration, and nonoperative management. Surg Obes Relat Dis. 2015;**11**:739-748

[76] Nimeri A, Ibrahim M, Maasher A, Al HM. Management Algorithm for Leaks Following Laparoscopic Sleeve Gastrectomy. Obes Surg. 2016;**26**:21-25

[77] Souto-Rodríguez R, Alvarez-Sánchez M-V. Endoluminal solutions to bariatric surgery complications: A review with a focus on technical

aspects and results. World J Gastrointest Endosc. 2017;**9**:**105**-126

[78] Parikh A, Alley JB, Peterson RM, et al. Management options for symptomatic stenosis after laparoscopic vertical sleeve gastrectomy in the morbidly obese. Surg Endosc. 2012;**26**:738-746

[79] Shnell M, Fishman S, Eldar S, Goitein D, Santo E. Balloon dilatation for symptomatic gastric sleeve stricture. Gastrointest Endosc. 2014;**79**:521-524

[80] Kalaiselvan R, Ammori BJ. Laparoscopic median gastrectomy for stenosis following sleeve gastrectomy. Surg Obes Relat Dis. 2015;**11**:474-477

[81] Oor JE, Roks DJ, Ünlü Ç, Hazebroek EJ. Laparoscopic sleeve gastrectomy and gastroesophageal reflux disease: a systematic review and meta-analysis. Am J Surg. 2016;**211**:250-267

[82] Telem DA, Gould J, Pesta C, et al. American Society for Metabolic and Bariatric Surgery: care pathway for laparoscopic sleeve gastrectomy. Surg Obes Relat Dis. 2017;**13**:742-749

[83] Mandeville Y, Van Looveren R, Vancoillie P-J, et al. Moderating the Enthusiasm of Sleeve Gastrectomy: Up to Fifty Percent of Reflux Symptoms After Ten Years in a Consecutive Series of One Hundred Laparoscopic Sleeve Gastrectomies. Obes Surg. 2017;**27**:1797-1803

[84] Tan SBM, Greenslade J, Martin D, Talbot M, Loi K, Hopkins G. Portomesenteric vein thrombosis in sleeve gastrectomy: a 10-year review. Surg Obes Relat Dis. 2018;**14**:271-275

[85] Sarker A, Meek CL, Park A. Biochemical consequences of bariatric surgery for extreme clinical obesity. Ann Clin Biochem. 2016;**53**:21-31

[86] Gehrer S, Kern B, Peters T, Christoffel-Courtin C, Peterli R. Fewer nutrient deficiencies after laparoscopic sleeve gastrectomy (LSG) than after laparoscopic Roux-Y-gastric bypass (LRYGB)-a prospective study. Obes Surg. 2010;**20**:447-453

[87] Hutter MM, Schirmer BD, Jones DB, et al. First report from the American College of Surgeons Bariatric Surgery Center Network: laparoscopic sleeve gastrectomy has morbidity and effectiveness positioned between the band and the bypass. Ann Surg. 2011;**254**:410-420 discussion 420-422

Chapter 7

Sleeve-Plus Procedures in Asia: Duodenojejunal Bypass and Proximal Jejunal Bypass

Michelle Bernadette C. Lim-Loo, Chih-Kun Huang, Valerie Chan and Kathleen Chua

Abstract

Laparoscopic sleeve gastrectomy (SG) is the most commonly done bariatric procedure worldwide due to its technical ease. However, the physiologic effects of this procedure have limitations on glucose homeostasis for patients with type 2 Diabetes Mellitus (T2DM). This is due to the insufficient physiologic modulations from intestinal hormones. The Roux-en-Y gastric bypass (RYGB) has been proven to have better T2DM remission than SG due to more pronounced physiologic changes from foregut and hindgut hormone modulations. However, RYGB is technically challenging to perform and is accompanied by many potential postoperative complications, especially in terms of nutrition. The addition of an intestinal bypass to SG also induces said intestinal hormone changes to enhance diabetes remission. This chapter discusses the intestinal bypass that may be added to SG as surgical options for the treatment of obesity and T2DM with focus on duodenojejunal and proximal jejunal bypass.

Keywords: sleeve gastrectomy with bypass, sleeve-plus, duodenojejunal bypass, proximal jejunal bypass, morbid obesity, type 2 diabetes, bariatric surgery in Asia

1. Introduction

Obesity rates continue to increase globally, as well as the number of bariatric surgeries done. The RYGB is considered the gold standard bariatric surgery due to its satisfactory weight loss and remission of T2DM and other morbidities. However, the technical complexity and its long-term complications have led to a decrease in popularity over SG, which is easier to do with also satisfactory outcomes in weight loss and resolution of morbidities. However, SG also has its own shortcomings such as long-term weight regains and recurrence of co-morbidities. In an attempt to improve outcomes and decrease complications, new procedures are developed. Supplementing an intestinal bypass to an SG results in a simpler technique that has the physiologic advantages of RYGB but minimized adverse effects. The term for such procedures was coined as "sleeve-plus" by Dr. Chih-Kun Huang in the Taiwan Surgical Society of Gastroenterology meeting on October 24, 2015 [1]. As there have been several types of sleeve-plus techniques, this chapter will give a more comprehensive discussion on sleeve-plus procedures more commonly done in the Asia-Pacific region: the duodeno-jejunal bypass (DJB) and the proximal jejunal bypass (PJB).

2. World statistics and census

Obesity is a major non-communicable epidemic disease and has been increasing worldwide for both developed and developing countries. It has tripled in number since 1975 according to the World Health Organization (WHO), with the latest data showing more than 1.9 billion adults classified as overweight; 650 million of which are considered as obese. In 2016, obesity accounted for 13% of the world's population (11% of men, 15% of women) [2]. In the Asia-Pacific region, the obesity in Gulf countries is greater than 30%, with T2DM frequency at 8-14.7%. This is in contrast to most of the other Asian countries where diabetes was more frequently seen than obesity [3].

Bariatric surgery is recognized as the most efficacious treatment for morbid obesity and its accompanying co-morbidities [4]. The International Federation for the Surgery of Obesity and Metabolic Disorders (IFSO) 5th Global Registry Report in 2019 recorded 520,983 bariatric operations performed from 2015 to 2018. The predominating bariatric surgery was SG (58.6%) followed by RYGB (31.6%) [5]. The Asia-Pacific Bariatric and Metabolic Surgery Society 2018 Congress reported 95,125 surgeries in Asia-Pacific countries, with most being performed in Australia and the Gulf countries, reflecting the highest obese populations in Asia. The most commonly performed was SG (68%), followed by the different bypass procedures (19.5%), and other surgeries, including revisional surgery (12.5%). Sleeve gastrectomy is being done at more than 50% of the procedures in most countries. The reported bypass surgeries included RYGB, one-anastomosis gastric bypass, SG with duodenojejunal bypass (SGDJB), and biliopancreatic duodenal switch (BPPDS). The bypass procedures were more than 30% only in Thailand and India. The OAGB was the leading bypass procedure in Taiwan, India and the Gulf countries. The SGDJB was more common in Japan, while RYGB was more common in the other countries [3].

The gold standard in bariatric surgery is still RYGB; but due to its technical difficulty and more severe complications such as marked malnutrition and marginal ulceration, SG has become the more popular bariatric procedure.

3. Brief evolution of bariatric surgery

Bariatric and metabolic surgery originated in the early 1950s, first performed by Kremen: the jejunoileal bypass. To treat obesity-associated hyperlipidemia, the proximal jejunum was anastomosed to the distal ileum to limit absorption. However, this was associated with post-operative severe malnutrition and liver complications [6]. Taiwan was the first country in Asia recorded to perform the jejunoileal bypass for obesity treatment in 1974 [7]. The initial bariatric surgery was modified to limit malabsorption. In 1960s, Mason developed the first gastric bypass procedure utilizing a transverse gastric pouch remnant anastomosed to a loop of jejunum. Severe bile reflux prompted revision to a Roux-en-Y reconstruction of gastric bypass in the 1970s, which resulted to less diarrhea, kidney stones and gallbladder stones [6]. Taiwan was the first to perform a gastric partition in 1981. Vertical banded gastroplasty then began in Japan in 1982, and then Singapore in 1987 [7].

Biliopancreatic diversion (BPD) by Scopinario and duodenal switch (DS) by Hess were also developed subsequently in 1976 and 1988; but the high incidence of potential metabolic complications and prolonged follow-up made these procedures less common. The RYGB eventually became the gold standard procedure for bariatric surgery [4].

In an attempt to breakdown RYGB and laparoscopic DS to decrease the operative time, SG was initially performed as a first step of a staged procedure [8]. The achievement of weight loss after SG made it an adequate stand-alone procedure.

Laparoscopic bariatric surgeries were first performed in 1994: laparoscopic adjustable gastric banding (LAGB) by Belachaew, and laparoscopic RYGB by Wittgrove and Clark. Asia also started laparoscopic bariatric surgeries during the 1990s [3]. In 1999, laparoscopic BPDDS was initiated by Gagner; and laparoscopic classical BPD by Scopinario. By 2000, McMahon and Gagner performed the first isolated laparoscopic SG, which was the time that majority of bariatric surgeries were already being done laparoscopically [5, 9].

Advancements in minimally invasive surgery lead to the application of single incision laparoscopic surgery (SILS) to bariatric surgery. In 2008, Nguyen reported the first case of bariatric SILS with adjustable gastric banding, [10] while Saber performed SILS SG [11]. Huang documented the first single incision transumbilical (SITU) RYGB in 2009, [12] followed by a series in 2010 comparing surgical outcomes of patients undergoing 5-port LRYGB with the novel SITU RYGB. The SILS has been shown to improve patient satisfaction in terms of cosmesis with comparable weight loss and morbidity rate. However, technical challenges due to the restricted surgical field, longer operative time, and increased post-operative pain have limited its popularity [13]. These procedures are technically feasible and reproducible with proper patient selection, performed by an experienced surgeon.

Restrictive and malabsorptive anatomic conceptualization of bariatric surgical procedures are continually under investigation. Modifications to the accepted standards are being made to further improve the treatment of obesity-related co-morbidities and reduce the impact of surgery.

4. Types of sleeve-plus procedures

The earliest sleeve-plus procedure is the BPDDS which was developed in 1998 by Hess and Marceau [14, 15]. Many of the sleeve plus procedures were patterned after the BPDDS. The procedure consists of a Roux-en-Y reconstruction of the bowel with a duodeno-ileal anastomosis for the alimentary limb, a lengthy biliopancreatic limb for malabsorption, and a short common limb. Changes in the location of the limb anastomosis and the limb lengths resulted in the different sleeve-plus techniques reported today (**Figure 1**).

In 2007, Sanchez-Pernaute reported a modification of the BPDDS into a loop fashion of limb reconstruction with a longer common channel. He described it as a single anastomosis duodenoileal bypass with sleeve (SADI-S) [16]. Santoro developed the SG with transit bipartition as an ileal anastomosis to the SG antrum with a Roux-en-Y reconstruction. This technique was then revised by Mui into a loop fashion and was called single anastomosis sleeve ileal bypass (SASI) [17, 18].

The sleeve gastrectomy duodenojejunal bypass (SGDJB) was first developed in Asia as an alternative to RYGB to allow the stomach to be screened for gastric cancer in areas with a high-risk population. The procedure may be done in the Roux-en-Y or loop fashion and was developed by Kasama in Japan and Huang in Taiwan, respectively [19, 20].

The ileal interposition with sleeve gastrectomy (IISG) was introduced by Aureo De Paula. The procedure included a segment of the ileum placed between the transected proximal duodenum and to the proximal jejunum, or interposed into the proximal jejunum [21]. The complexity of the procedure limits its widespread application.

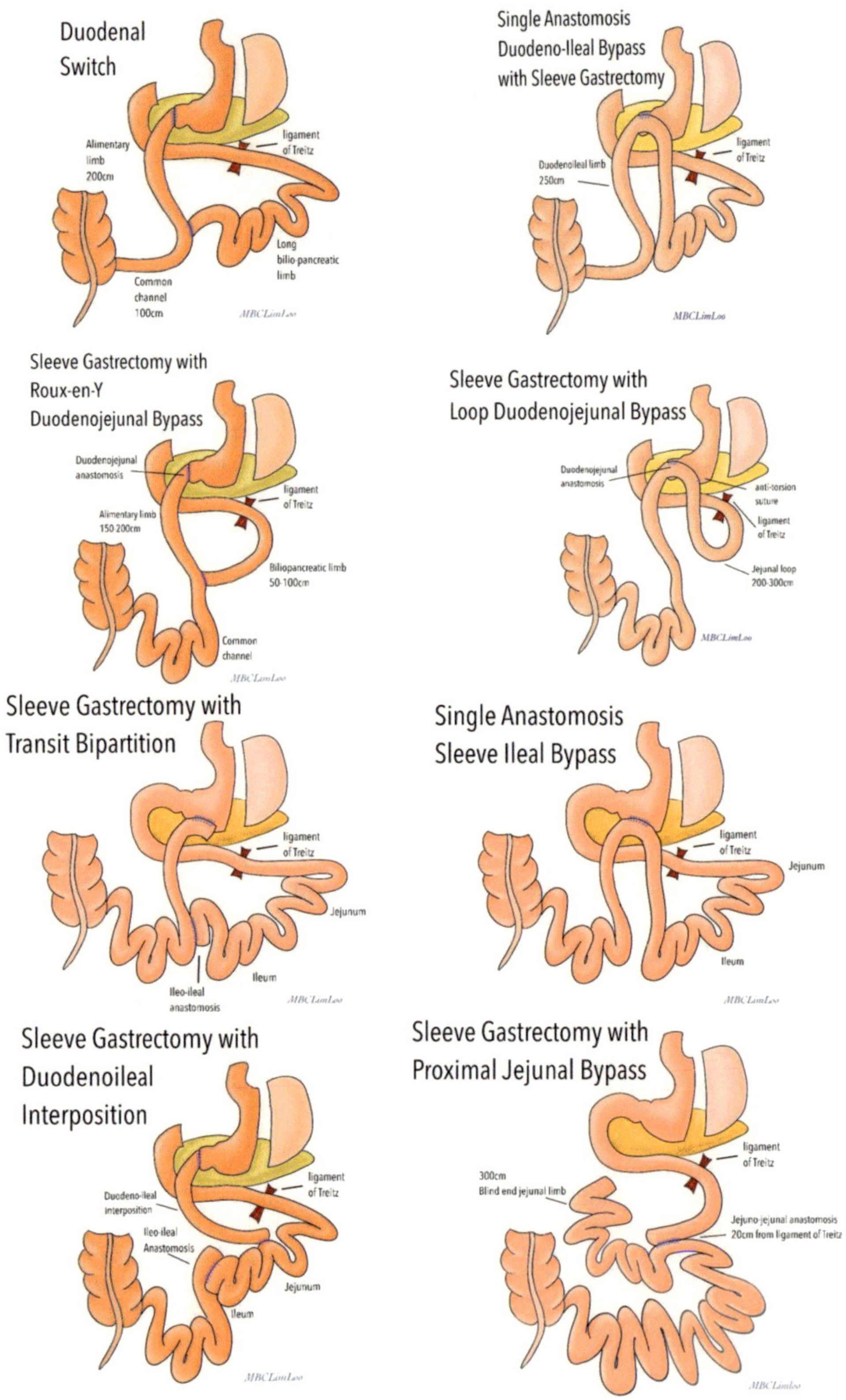

Figure 1.
Types of sleeve-plus procedures.

The proximal jejunal bypass (SGPJB) is probably the simplest sleeve-plus procedure to perform. It was developed by Alamo in 2004, where the proximal 20 cm of the jejunum is transected and anastomosed to the distal 300 cm bowel, leaving a blind-ended segment of the jejunum [22].

5. Advantages of sleeve-plus procedures

Several advantages can be gained from sleeve-plus procedures. First, it allows the remaining stomach to be screened for gastric cancer, which is frequently done in areas of high gastric cancer prevalence such as Japan and Korea [23]. Screening will be difficult to do in RYGB.

In the techniques where anatomical and functional preservation of the pylorus is done, the gastric mucosa is protected against pancreatic and biliary fluids; hence, preventing bile acid gastritis [24]. The pylorus also regulates gastric emptying which results to a lower incidence of dumping syndrome [25]. The larger gastric mucosal contact to food in SG compared to that in RYGB also improves the absorption of iron, calcium, vitamin B_{12} and protein leading to less nutritional deficiencies [26].

Sleeve-plus procedures are quite versatile if a conversion to another procedure become warranted, whether due to weight regain, or complications of leaks and strictures. The loop SGDJB may be converted to a DS by transecting the afferent limb and anastomosing it to the distal segment of the efferent limb. The Roux-en-Y SGDJB can also be converted into DS by lengthening the alimentary limb from the biliopancreatic limb. Conversion to RYGB of any sleeve-plus procedure is also feasible. Index sleeve-plus procedures with a transected duodenum requires the proximal duodenal anastomosis to be taken down to allow resection of the distal gastric tube. The previous alimentary limb is then anastomosed to the remaining gastric pouch. In an SGPJB, a gastric pouch is simply created and anastomosed to the blind limb to construct the alimentary limb. In SG with bipartition, the gastroenteric anastomosis is transected, a gastric pouch is created, and a Roux-en-Y reconstruction of the bowel is done.

Loop techniques of sleeve-plus procedures have an additional advantage over the Roux-en-Y techniques. The single anastomosis in loop procedures allow for a shorter operative time and less potential complications that may arise from every additional anastomosis. The number of anastomoses also translates to the number of man-made hernial defects that necessitates closure. Another advantage of the loop techniques is that marginal ulcers have not been reported [20]. This may be due to the immediate neutralization of the gastric fluid by the bile juices once in the duodenum.

6. Hormonal effect of sleeve-plus procedures

When food is ingested, there are changes in the entero-insular axis which involve the gastrointestinal, endocrine and pancreatic secretions that contribute to insulin production. The main hormones in this mechanism includes ghrelin, glucagon-like polypeptide (GLP-1), peptide YY (PYY), gastric inhibitory peptide, oxyntomodulin, and cholecystokinin. Anatomical alterations of the food passageway can affect these entero-hormones which can both influence the central regulation of body weight homeostasis, and make glycemic control more efficient. The hormones affect the hypothalamic-appetite regulation and suppress food intake. The enhanced glucose homeostasis can be explained by "foregut" and "hindgut" theories. The foregut theory hypothesizes that exclusion of food contact with the duodenum prevents secretion of "anti-incretin" substances. Incretins are metabolic hormones that promote a decrease in blood glucose by making the pancreas more efficient. On the other hand, the hindgut theory explains that contact of undigested food immediately into the distal bowel stimulates production of incretins. The more relevant incretins involved are the GLP-1 and the PYY. These are produced from the L-cells in the distal ileum and colon after immediate contact with nutrients. The postprandial GLP-1 levels are significantly increased after both RYGB and LSG [27–29].

The sleeve-plus procedures are comprised of a sleeve gastrectomy and an intestinal bypass component. Sleeve gastrectomy has been shown to significantly decrease ghrelin, an orexigenic hormone predominantly secreted in the stomach. Ghrelin is also known to suppress insulin and have a modulating effect on glucose homeostasis, hence the decreased levels after SG also helps improve blood sugar control [30]. The SGPJB and SGDJB both have additional glycemic control effect by allowing food to be in early contact to the distal jejunum, stimulating earlier incretin production. The SGDJB has the added benefit of bypassing the duodenum and averts secretion of anti-incretin substances [31].

6.1 Hormonal study

A prospective observational study was conducted by Dr. Chih-Kun Huang on the incretin effect of SGDJB in type II diabetic patients with BMI <35 kg/m^2 from May 2013 to March 2014. The study included 27 patients, 23 females and four males, mean age of 51, mean weight at 74.5 kg and mean BMI 28.4 kg/m^2. All patients have T2DM for a mean duration of 10 years and underwent SGDJB with an afferent limb of 200 cm. The C-peptide, ghrelin, GLP-1, PYY were measured over time together with an oral glucose tolerance test (OGTT).

Hormone levels were analyzed by time courses, area under the plasma concentration time profile (AUC) and maximum plasma concentration (Cmax). Follow-up hormone levels were compared using the paired t-test. The fisher exact test was used when 20% of the cells had expected values of less than 5. A p-value of less than 0.05 denoted statistical significance. All statistical tests were 2-tailed and calculated using the SPSS statistical software (version 15.0; SPSS Inc., Chicago Il.)

The surgery resulted in substantial weight loss with good glycemic control. At six months, the mean BMI had decreased to 22 ($p < 0.01$), fasting glucose from 160 to 111 gm/dL, and mean glycosylated hemoglobin levels from 9.3 to 6.28% ($p < 0.01$). Fasting ghrelin assays over time alongside OGTT was significantly lower with an AUC-120 of 82.13 ± 49.36 pg./mL/min dropping down to 17.90 ± 9.01 pg./mL/min ($p < 0.05$). The GLP-1 showed an exaggerated response with an AUC-120 increase from 139.37 ± 109.93 pg./mL/min preoperatively to 349.10 ± 187.35 pg./mL/min at one month ($p < 0.05$) and to 185.75 ± 118.81 pg./mL/min at six months ($p = 0.06$). The PYY also showed significant postprandial response at one month postoperatively with and AUC-120 change from 137.10 ± 93.20 pg./mL/min to 454.50 ± 134.85 pg./mL/min ($p < 0.05$). However, this dropped to 136.57 ± 134.53 pg./mL/min at six months ($p = 0.987$) postoperatively (**Figure 2**).

The results in this hormonal study can infer that SGDJB leads to the immediate decrease in hunger, increase in satiety and better glycemic control. However, the decrease in PYY levels after six months is different from that of other hormonal studies where GLP-1 and PYY were shown to be elevated up to one year after bariatric surgery [32, 33]. Further research is needed to confirm how long the elevated incretin levels can persist postoperatively and how the body eventually adapts to it.

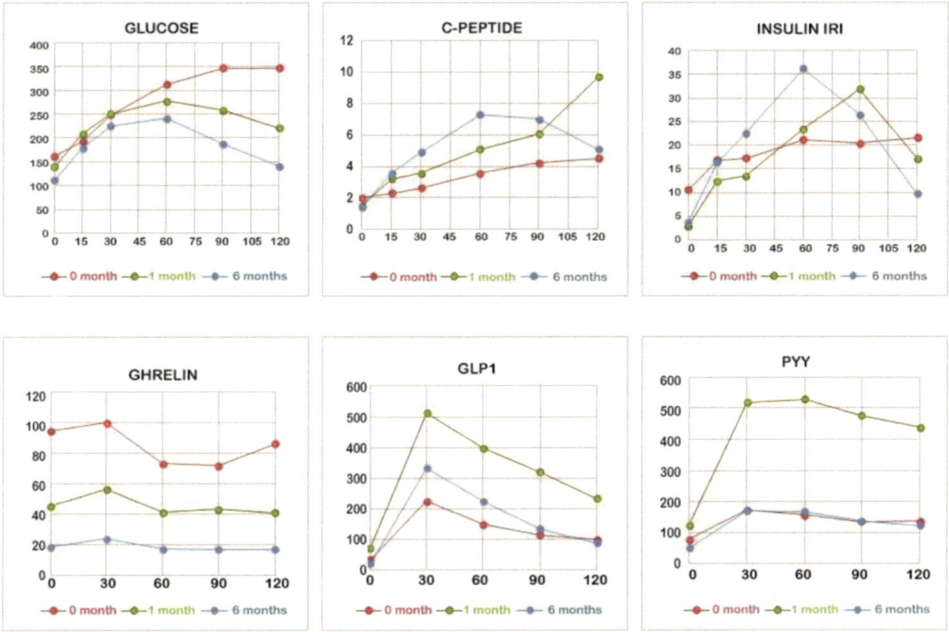

Figure 2.
C-peptide and hormone assays at zero, one and six months after SGDJB against time in minutes alongside an oral glucose tolerance test.

7. Indications and contraindications

The National Institute of Health (NIH) Consensus Conference in 1991 established the indications in performing bariatric surgery, at the height of the obesity epidemic. Since then, a few modifications were made differing from country to country. The National Institute of Health and Care Excellence (NICE) in UK, as well as the Asian Pacific Metabolic and Bariatric Surgery Society (APMBSS), extended the indications further in relation to presence of other co-morbidities and adjusted the BMI threshold in accordance to inherent differences in body composition [34, 35]. In 2016, the 2nd Diabetes Surgery Summit convened with leading international diabetes organizations and developed new recommendations for metabolic surgery with a lower BMI threshold for Asians due to the higher risk for diabetes despite lower BMI values [36, 37] (**Table 1**).

Contraindications to bariatric surgery include physiological, medical and surgical, and psychological factors; few are considered to be absolute contraindications (**Table 2**).

Physiological factors include age and BMI. Initial NIH guidelines have limited surgery to 18-65 years of age, but recent studies have shown that bariatric surgery is considered safe for the elderly population [38–41]. There are limited well-designed prospective studies on bariatric surgery for children and adolescents, and an important factor to take into consideration is the psychological maturity required in accepting the lifestyle changes accompanying surgical intervention.

Obstructive sleep apnea, diabetes, hypertension and cardiovascular problems are some of the health conditions that should be screened and controlled preoperatively prior to contemplating bariatric surgery. Previous abdominal surgery including abdominal wall hernias would influence practicality and applicability of any laparoscopic approach [4].

Criteria	NIH	NICE	APMBSS	DSS-II[i]
BMI	≥ 40	≥ 40	> 37	≥ 40[i]
BMI with co-morbidities	≥35-	• ≥ 35 • ≥ 35 with new onset diabetes • 30 with new onset diabetes*	≥ 32**	• ≥35[i]*** • ≥30[i]****

[i]BMI criteria is decreased by 2.5 for Asians.
**Bariatric surgery can be considered in BMI 30-34.9 with new onset diabetes.*
***Presence of diabetes or two other obesity-related co-morbidities.*
****Inadequately controlled hyperglycemia despite lifestyle and optimal medical therapy.*
*****Inadequately controlled hyperglycemia despite optimal medical treatment.*

Table 1.
Indications for bariatric surgery.

Absolute Contraindications
Poor functional status Uncontrollable psychiatric disease Drug or substance abuse Malignancy
Relative Contraindications
Extremes of age Type 1 Diabetes Mellitus Smoking Liver cirrhosis Previous abdominal surgery

Table 2.
Contraindications for bariatric surgery.

Active psychiatric disease and psychological instability are absolute contraindications; while poorly controlled eating disorders being a negative predictor of post-operative weight loss, is a relative contraindication [42, 43]. Smoking has been associated with development of post-operative marginal ulceration after gastric bypass, increased risk of poor wound healing and impaired health, and should be stopped at least 6 weeks before surgery [4, 44].

7.1 Selection of sleeve-plus procedure

The SGDJB and SGPJB are both relatively more recent than the RYGB and the data is still too young to provide specific indications for either procedures. Both patient and surgical factors must be considered when choosing the appropriate procedure for a safe outcome with optimal weight loss and resolution of co-morbidities. Any contraindications to SG obviously preclude both SGDJB and SGPJB such as severe gastroesophageal reflux disease and Barrett's esophagus.

All patients who are suitable candidates for SG may benefit from an additional bypass component if the BMI and diabetic history are considered. Higher BMIs such as 45 or more may benefit from a malabsorptive component but also reflect thicker visceral fat. This may pose difficulties during duodenal dissection for SGDJB. Hence, SGPJB may be a safer and easier option. Patients with long standing diabetes may also benefit from a bypass component because of the additional incretin response. Those with poorer glycemic control due to a more decompensated pancreas may consider SGDJB over SGPJB due to the combined glycemic effects from the foregut and hindgut theory. However, SGDJB is a challenging procedure and requires a more experienced surgeon's skill set.

Intraoperative findings may also influence the choice of procedure. Any evidence of vascular perfusion concerns on otherwise normal tissues may hint potential anastomotic problems. An SGPJB may be a more practical option, as the leaks from jejuno-jejunal anastomosis is easier to manage than leaks from a duodenojejunal anastomosis. The patient's current medical condition must also be considered. Severe co-morbidities such as cardiac issues may preclude contemplation for SGDJB as this requires a longer operative time compared to SGPJB.

Each surgery has its own advantages and disadvantages. However, a safe outcome is still the most important factor to consider when choosing not only between sleeve-plus procedures, but for any type of bariatric surgery.

8. Preoperative considerations

A multidisciplinary team is necessary for screening and evaluating a patient's medical condition including psychological capability to undergo bariatric surgery. One of the crucial facets in the success of bariatric surgery is a comprehensive medical history, physical examination, preoperative work-up, with patient education playing an integral part.

A complete history should include a detailed diet history, physical activity, medication review, social history, psychological history, and psychosocial factors that can affect the surgical outcome. All body systems are assessed. A full endocrinologic evaluation is done to rule out other causes of obesity. Other obesity-related co-morbidities are screened and managed accordingly.

Psychological evaluation is necessary to identify any undiagnosed psychiatric disorders, and to assess if a candidate will be able to undergo the lifestyle changes necessary to sustain long-term weight loss. Any significant psychiatric problems must be treated and controlled prior to any contemplated procedure. Counseling for smoking and alcohol cessation, as well as pregnancy must be included.

9. Operative technique

The addition of a bypass component to a simple SG would entail a more technically challenging surgery. Advanced laparoscopic skills are essential to safely perform organ manipulations, adequate dissection, landmark identifications, suturing and anastomosis to ensure a complete and successful surgery. Although several procedures are mentioned above, this chapter will give a more comprehensive discussion to SGDJB and SGPJB, which are the more commonly performed sleeve-plus procedures in the Asia-Pacific region.

9.1 Duodenojejunal bypass

There have been two operative techniques describing SGDJB: the Roux-en-Y (RNY) and the loop technique. The RNY SGDJB was first described by Kasama in 2009 as an alternative option to RYGB which precludes screening of the remnant stomach for gastric cancer in high-risk populations as in Japan [19]. The loop technique was then described by Huang in 2013 in an attempt to mitigate some long-term complications associated with RYGB [20].

9.1.1 Roux-en-Y technique

After induction of anesthesia, the patient is placed in the French position. Five ports are inserted, the camera port at the supra-umbilicus, a 5-mm port at the subxiphoid for liver retraction, two 12-mm ports at the left subcostal margin and 10 cm caudally, and a 15 mm port at the right upper abdomen.

A standard SG is done over a 36 French bougie using linear staplers beginning 4 cm from the pylorus and proceeding proximally. Dissection of the posterior wall of the duodenum is done and transected at 1-2 cm distal to the pylorus. The jejunum is transected at 50-100 cm from the ligament of Treitz serving as the biliopancreatic limb. The transected distal jejunum to serve as the alimentary tract is measured to 150-200 cm where the jejunojejunostomy anastomosis of the biliopancreatic limb is done. The mesenteric defect is closed by hand-sewn technique. The omentum is divided to avoid tension on the antecolic reconstruction of the duodenojejunal end-to-side anastomosis [19] (**Figure 3**).

9.1.2 Loop technique

After anesthesia is initiated, the patient is placed in supine position. Five ports are also used. Two 12-mm ports at the left and right of the umbilicus at the midclavicular line; the left serving as the camera port. A 15-mm port is inserted into the umbilicus and two 5-mm ports at both subcostal margins.

A standard sleeve gastrectomy is done over a 36 French bougie using a linear stapler beginning at 4 cm proximal to the pylorus and proceeding cranially. At the duodenum 2 cm distal to the pylorus, the posterior wall is dissected creating a tunnel where the linear stapler is inserted and used for transection. The jejunum is then measured 200-300 cm from the Ligament of Treitz where an enterotomy is created. A 1.5 cm duodenotomy is created at the proximal limb and anastomosed to the enterotomy by hand-sewn technique. The jejunum 4 cm proximal to the duodenojejunostomy is anchored to the antrum serving as an anti-torsion suture. The Petersen's defect is closed. The remnant stomach is fixed posteriorly to the retroperitoneal fat and a Jackson-Pratt drain is placed behind the duodenojejunal anastomosis [20] (**Figure 4**).

9.1.3 Pearls

The SGDJB can be quite intimidating to some surgeons due to the intimate relationship of the duodenum to the surrounding structures. Proper identification of landmarks to guide dissection is important to avoid mishaps.

The location of the common bile duct running behind the first portion of the duodenum, serves as a boundary to the second portion where the transection is done. The gastroduodenal artery (GDA) is also located in this area just to the left of the common bile duct (**Figure 5**). Hence, dissection of the duodenum from the pancreas must be done carefully to avoid injury and bleeding due to the proximity of the GDA and high vascularity of the area.

To facilitate the dissection, counter-traction of the duodenum may be done by pulling the stomach laterally to the left using a traction suture over the gastric antrum. In patients with excessive periduodenal fat, the dissection of a tunnel below the duodenum becomes difficult. In these cases, the right gastroepiploic vessels may be sacrificed. Once a clear tunnel between the duodenum and pancreas has been created, a vascular tape may be inserted and used to lift the duodenum to assist insertion of a stapler for the duodenal transection (**Figure 6**). The surgeon must take care not to injure the common bile duct, pancreas and vasculatures around the first part of the duodenum. A side-to-side or end-to side duodenojejunal

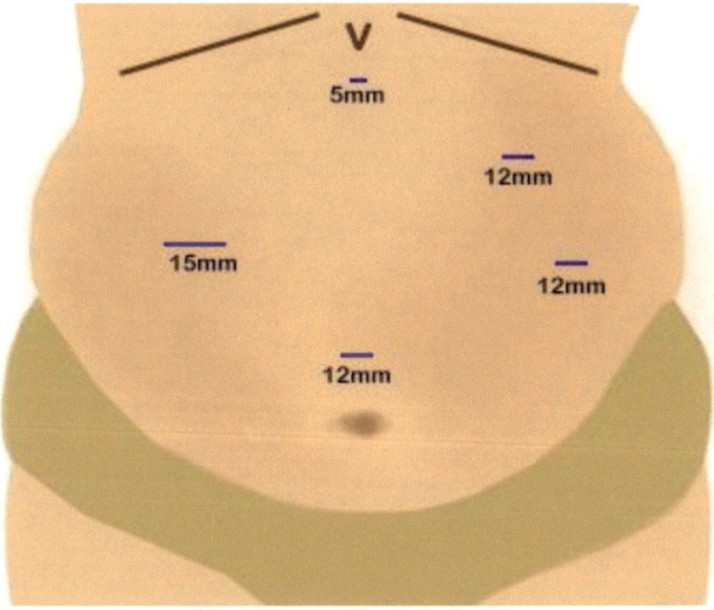

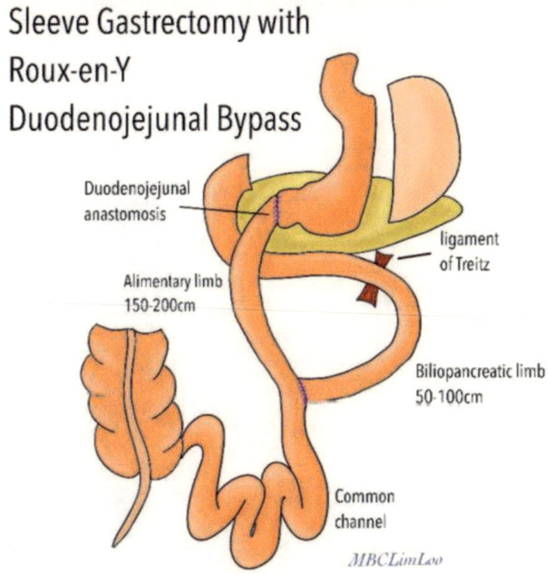

Figure 3.
SGDJB roux-en-Y technique.

anastomosis may be done, each having its own precautions. A side-to-side anastomosis must be done 1 cm distal to the pylorus to avoid its injury. A temporary stay suture between the pylorus and proximal jejunum allows for easier hand-sewn anastomosis. The other option of an end-to-side anastomosis would require the posterior wall of the proximal duodenum to be partially devascularized to allow some tissue clearance for the hand-sewn anastomosis. Use of a stapler in both orientation of anastomosis may risk pyloric injury. The loop technique requires only a single anastomosis, and an anti-torsion suture anchoring afferent limb of the jejunal loop to the stomach. This is done to avoid torsion or kinking of the jejunal limbs. The RNY technique would require another entero-enteric anastomosis which would translate to more operative time. Closure of both the Petersen and mesenteric defect prevents potential internal herniation of bowel.

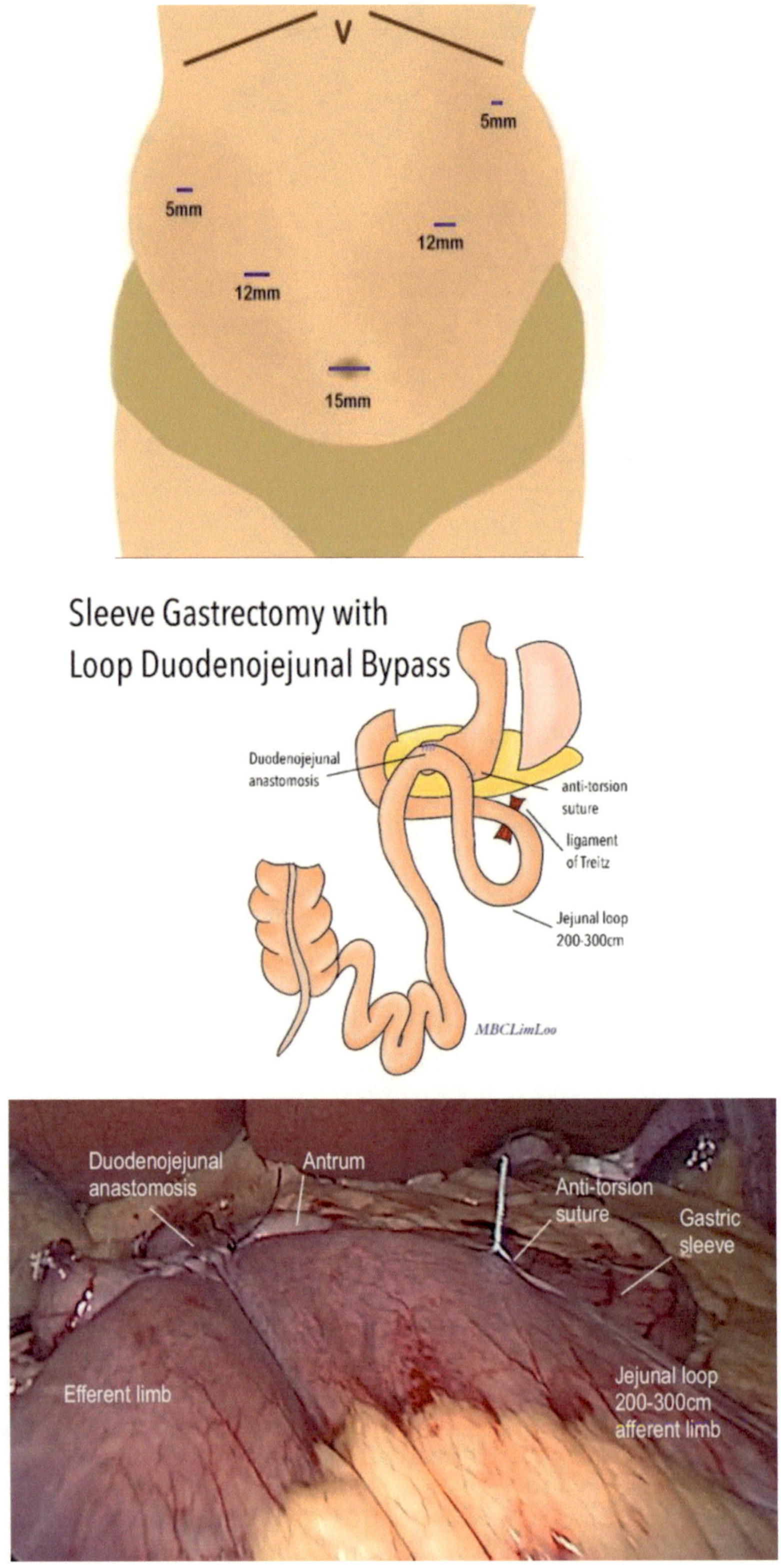

Figure 4.
SGDJB loop technique.

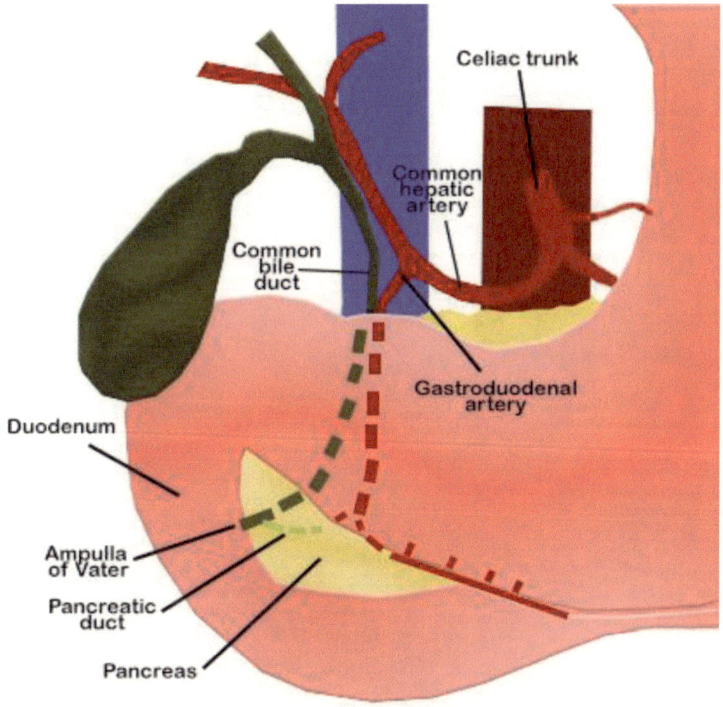

Figure 5.
Anatomical landmarks and relationships of the proximal duodenum.

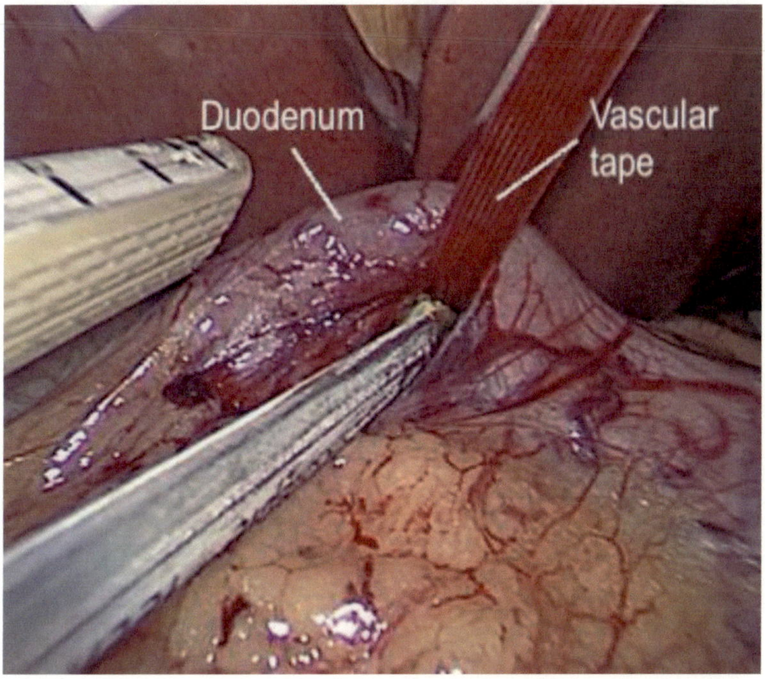

Figure 6.
Use of a vascular tape to maneuver the duodenum facilitates application of the stapling device.

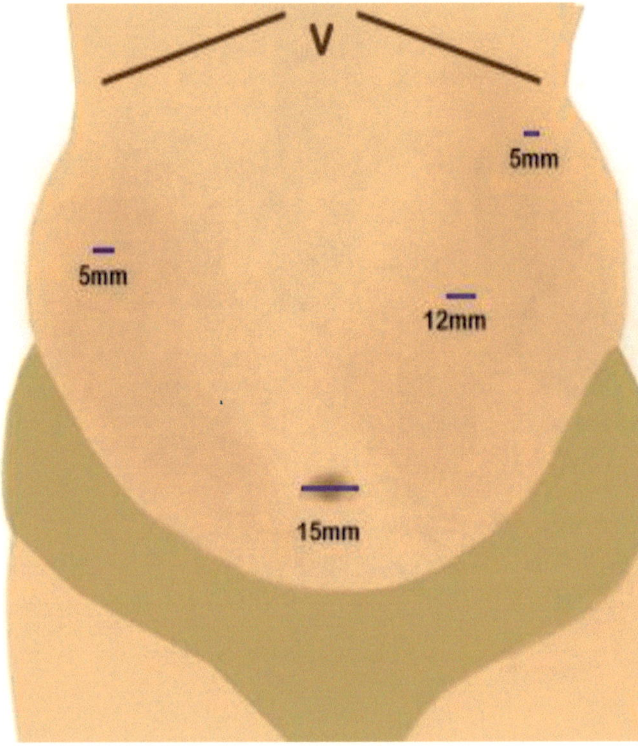

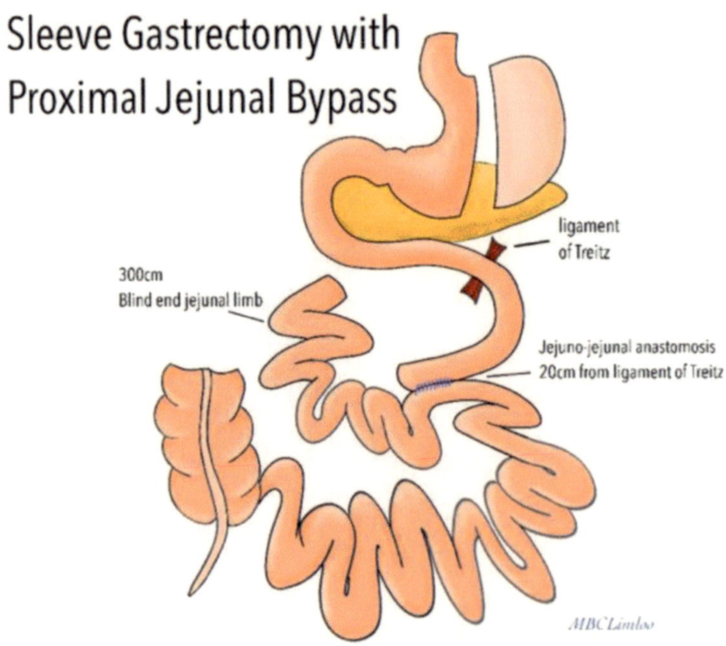

Figure 7.
Sleeve gastrectomy with proximal jejunal bypass.

9.1.4 Challenges

Apart from being an irreversible procedure with no long-term data available yet to compare it to RYGB, the procedure is technically demanding and might preclude super obese patients. It also requires a fastidious surgeon with meticulous skills in manipulating an area of intimately-related vital structures, so as to have an uneventful surgery.

Duodenal dissection and manipulation must be done carefully to avoid inadvertent damage to the duodenal wall. Injury to the duodenum proximal to the dissection is resolved with the duodenojejunal anastomosis. But injury distal to the transection may result in a leak if not repaired properly.

Bile duct injury may occur if the duodenal transection is done too distally. Avulsions and lacerations are repaired over a T-tube inserted into the bile duct. Complete transections would require a biliary reconstruction.

Bleeding is not infrequent due to the vascularity around the proximal duodenum and may range from oozing to torrential. Oozing due to multiple small vessels is controlled with simple packing until hemostasis is achieved. Added manipulation is avoided to prevent more tissue injury and aggravate hemorrhage. Severe bleeding from an injured gastroduodenal artery may necessitate suture repair, ligation or conversion to an open laparotomy.

Another shortcoming of the SGDJB is the inaccessibility to the Ampulla of Vater for endoscopic management of biliary obstructions. Therefore, patients with cholelithiasis preoperatively are offered cholecystectomy concomitantly with the bariatric surgery or subsequently if it develops postoperatively, regardless of symptoms.

9.2 Proximal Jejunal bypass

The surgery is performed under general anesthesia with the patient in reverse Trendelenberg position. Initial entry and camera port is done along the left upper quadrant followed by the other working ports: 15 mm at the umbilicus, 5 mm at the right upper quadrant, and 5 mm at the left subcostal area.

A standard SG is done over a 36 French bougie using linear staplers beginning 4 cm from the pylorus and proceeding proximally. The ligament of Treitz is identified and jejunum is divided at 20 cm. The distally transected jejunum is measured to a distance varying from 250 to 300 cm and is anastomosed to the proximal biliopancreatic jejunal limb. The mesenteric defect is closed to avoid internal hernia and the remnant stomach is fixed posteriorly to the retroperitoneal fat [15] (**Figure 7**).

10. Postoperative care and follow up

Once the surgery has been concluded, extubated and recovered from anesthesia, the patient is then returned to the ward. Clear liquids are initiated once the patient is fully awake. Deep breathing exercises and chest physiotherapy are done. Early mobilization is encouraged and opioid analgesics are used for pain control. If there are no remarkable events, the patient is discharged and is scheduled to follow up after one week at the out-patient clinic. Diet progression is then continued as with any routine bariatric diet, with a progressive exercise program in place. Maintenance medications for diabetes and other co-morbidities are adjusted accordingly. Prophylactic proton pump inhibitors may be given. Subsequent follow-ups include dietary counseling, and is done every three months after the surgery for the first two years and then annually.

11. Therapeutic outcomes

Review of literature has reported RYGB to have better results than LSG in terms of weight loss and T2DM remission. However, complications are also reported to be higher after RYGB [46, 47]. Up to 97% of morbidly obese SG patients have been reported to have improvement or remission of T2DM at 13 months but drops to 60.8% at five years with a recurrence rate of 13% [48]. Early reports of DJB in non-obese diabetic patients have shown improvement in sugar control albeit without remission of diabetes [49, 50]. Since there was no SG done, this suggests that weight loss is a strong factor for diabetes remission. The combination of SG with an intestinal bypass results to a synergistic combination of weight loss and sugar control.

The SGDJB was first reported by Kasama et al. in 2009, in comparison with gastric band, RYGB and SG. At one year, the excess weight loss (EWL) was similar to RYGB, and better than SG or gastric banding. Diabetes resolution of SGDJB was better than SG at 93% versus 67%. There was also resolution of dyslipidemia (100%) and hypertension (85.7%) [19]. Raj et al. published a randomized controlled trial between SGDJB and RYGB showing no statistical difference in percent EWL, diabetes remission, and resolution of hypertension and dyslipidemia [51]. Lee et al. also compared SGDJB with RYGB showing better EWL with SGDJB (80.3% vs. 63.4%) but with higher cholesterol levels than RYGB [26]. He also compared SGDJB to SG alone and reported SGDJB to have better weight loss (EWL 87.2% versus 67.5%) and diabetes remission (93% versus 87%) [52].

Kasama's group also reported the effect of SGDJB on glucose metabolism in morbid obesity with associated diabetes. Glucose monitoring showed decreasing insulin requirements on the first postoperative day to no diabetic medications on the second day. At one month, 91% of the subjects achieved an HbA_1c below 7%. A meal tolerance test conducted at six months showed the subjects to have lower glucose and increased insulin area under the curve. This was reflected in the decreased requirement of oral hypoglycemic agents and insulin [53]. At one year, fasting blood sugar and HbA_1c levels improved at 194 to 105 and 8.9 to 6.0, respectively, and found to be sustained up to five years with a reported remission rate of 63.6% [54].

In diabetic patients within the lower BMI range of obesity, Huang et al. reported that SGDJB resulted in a BMI drop to 22.4 from 28.4 in six months, and HbA_1c levels below 7.0 without medications in 91% of the subjects [20]. On two-year follow-up, diabetes remission was found to be at 54% and glycemic control in 77% [55]. In comparison to RYGB, there were no statistical difference in the outcomes for diabetic patients with BMI less than 35 in terms of weight loss and glycemic control [56].

Studies on SGPJB have shown to the weight loss outcomes to be better than SG [57]. The EWL in one year is 96.7% and has been found to be sustained to more than 80% even after 10 years of follow-up [58]. Good glycemic control is also achieved after SGPJB. In 2016, the first Asian series was reported by Huang et al. showed 66% EWL at six months, with 66.7% of diabetic patients achieving an HbA_1c less than 6 without medications [45]. A study on diabetics with BMI of <35 showed 97% of the subjects on preoperative oral hypoglycemic agents had complete remission and all of the subjects on insulin to be in partial remission [59]. When compared with RYGB, the outcomes at one and three years showed weight loss and diabetes remission to be similar, with both groups requiring less medications [60, 61].

12. Complications

The overall morbidity associated with bariatric surgery complications ranges from 3.4-13% and may vary depending on the procedural type, surgical approach, patient age, BMI and co-morbidities [62–64]. Literature will show that SG has an overall complication rate lower than RYGB [65, 66]; however, potential complications associated with SG remains worrisome, including post-operative hemorrhage and staple line leak.

12.1 Hemorrhage

Significant post-operative hemorrhage after bariatric surgery has been described up to 3.4%, [67] with the most common presenting symptom as tachycardia (46%), followed by melena (32%). Sleeve gastrectomy bleeding can happen from the short gastric vessels or along the staple line after transection of the stomach [68]. Bleeding can also occur from an anastomotic site intraluminally in patients with an additional bypass procedure which typically may be managed medically or endoscopically. Surgery should be considered for hemodynamic instability and failure of endoscopic therapy [67].

12.2 Leak

One of the most dreaded complication after bariatric surgeries are anastomotic leaks or staple-line leaks. Leaks from SG can occur along the staple-line, with an average incidence of 1.5% [69]. Risk factors that contributed to gastrointestinal leak include oxygen dependency, hypoalbuminemia, sleep apnea, hypertension and diabetes. Additional factors that contributed to a higher leak rate include intraoperative provocative testing and placement of drain [70].

Clinical presentation of patients with leaks range from completely asymptomatic, to frank peritonitis, septic shock, and death. Unexplained tachycardia has been shown to be an initial sign of early leak [71]. Other potential signs that should cause a high index of suspicion should include fever (>38C), diffuse abdominal tenderness, cough, and persistent hiccups [72]. A concern about a leak should be investigated urgently with imaging modalities such as upper gastrointestinal series with water-soluble contrast or abdominal CT scan IV and oral contrast. Urgent reoperation is warranted for unstable patients with signs of sepsis. Stable patients with controlled leaks may undergo percutaneous drainage, antibiotic therapy and nutritional support, in conjunction with endoluminal therapies (stenting, clipping) [4, 72].

12.3 Sleeve gastrectomy related complications

12.3.1 Gastroesophageal reflux disease

Another SG related complication is new-onset gastroesophageal reflux disease (GERD), or worsening of previous GERD symptoms. A meta-analysis by Yeung et al. demonstrated significant worsening of GERD post-operatively at 19%, with de novo GERD at 23% [73]. Long-term follow up of patients show 28% of LSG patients develop esophagitis, and 8% develop Barrett's esophagus. Endoscopic assessment for presence of hiatal hernia is recommended pre-operatively, as its concomitant repair during SG can help reduce incidence of post-operative GERD [74].

12.3.2 Gastric tube stenosis

Post-SG stenosis is a rare complication with a reported incidence of 1% – 3.5% [75, 76]. The most common site for stenosis is at the incisura angularis, [76] usually presenting with gastric outlet obstruction symptoms with marked weight loss and malnutrition [4]. Diagnosis can be done with upper gastrointestinal series or contrast enhanced CT scan of the upper abdomen. Factors that contribute to development of stenosis include bougie size and oversewing of the staple line. Endoscopic dilatation is the first line of treatment which usually require multiple sessions. Failure of endoscopic intervention, long segment stenosis, or presence of delayed leakage, abscess or fistula formation necessitates surgical intervention [75, 76].

12.4 Intestinal bypass related complications

12.4.1 Hernia

Reconstruction of the intestinal continuity leads to man-made defects that may potentially result in internal hernias if not closed. Patients would present signs and symptoms of bowel obstruction and gangrene which are supported with radiologic findings. The incidence in SGDJB and SGPJB has been reported to be at 1-2% [51, 54, 60]. Despite the low incidence, defect closure still prevents the potential morbidities of internal hernia including necrosis and ischemia in 7-42% and associated mortalities [8].

Trocar site hernias are also a potential morbidity if facial defects more than 10 mm are not closed. When trocar sites where dilatated to allow extraction of specimens, this must also be closed [77].

12.4.2 Malnutrition

The addition of an intestinal bypass to sleeve gastrectomy has implications to the patient's nutritional status as it alters the natural absorption of nutrients. The larger stomach in sleeve-plus procedures allow more acid and intrinsic factors to have better absorption of iron, calcium, and vitamin B_{12} compared to an RYGB.

Comparison of SGDJB to SG alone has not shown any difference in nutritional status at one year [22, 52]. Investigational studies of SGDJB done in Chinese diabetic patients with BMI <25 kg/m^2 has shown an increased incidence of becoming underweight and deficiencies in iron, vitamin B_{12}, vitamin D and calcium [78].

In SGPJB, despite a defunctionalized intestinal segment, nutrient deficiency levels are comparable to SG. The preserved pyloric function and duodenal exclusion omitted in SGPJB also results to a lower incidence of nutritional deficiencies, diarrhea (6% vs. 21.5%), dumping syndrome (0 vs. 7.6%) and fatigue (25.3% vs. 40.5%) [61].

Postoperative supplementation of vitamins and minerals are necessary to prevent post-operative malnutrition. More studies are needed to determine the nutritional deficiency of sleeve-plus procedures to properly guide supplementation of these patients.

12.4.3 Dumping syndrome

Reconstruction of the digestive anatomy also alters the glucose metabolism which may result to dumping syndrome. This occurs in 15-76% after RYGB and may be potentially debilitating. Preservation of the pylorus in both SGDJB and SGPJB allows for a more regulated gastric emptying and a lower reported incidence of dumping syndrome at 4% and 0%, respectively [53, 61].

12.4.4 Marginal ulcer

Marginal ulcers of the gastrojejunal anastomosis of the RYGB has been reported to occur up to 12% and can lead to bleeding, perforation or stenosis. This is in contrast to low incidence reported in SGDJB Roux-en-Y technique at 0.49%, and no reported incidence in the loop technique [39, 54].

12.4.5 Blind loop syndrome

The creation of a blind loop of intestine could cause bacterial overgrowth, the so-called 'blind loop syndrome' or 'bacterial overgrowth syndrome' (BOS).

However, the SGPJB has the benefit of a blind jejunal limb without passage of food or bile, and an isoperistaltic loop [79]. This helps mitigate against the possibility of BOS. Unlike in JIB having a shorter common channel, the SGPJB enteral anastomosis has a longer common channel, in which bacterial concentration is significantly lower [60]. Incidence of BOS after SGPJB is still unknown, but intestine continuity can be easily reversed in case BOS develops.

13. Conclusion

The addition of a malabsorptive component to LSG has been coined as "sleeve-plus". The sleeve-plus procedures more commonly done in the Asia-Pacific are the SGDJB and SGPJB. The said procedures have both shown satisfactory outcomes in the treatment of obesity and related co-morbidities that are comparable to other bariatric procedures but with less adverse outcomes than that of RYGB and may be considered as alternative options. However, more studies are necessary to assess long-term outcomes in terms of diabetes remission, nutrition, and applicability to other racial populations.

Acknowledgements

The authors would like to thank Dr. Abhishek Katakwar for providing the data, statistical analysis and results of the hormonal study.

Conflict of interest

The authors declare that they have no competing interest.

Author details

Michelle Bernadette C. Lim-Loo[1]*, Chih-Kun Huang[2], Valerie Chan[1] and Kathleen Chua[1]

1 Chinese General Hospital and Medical Center, Manila, Philippines

2 Body science and Metabolic disorders International Medical Center, China Medical University Hospital, Taichung, Taiwan

*Address all correspondence to: docmichlim@gmail.com

References

[1] Huang CK, Liu CC, Hsin MC, Chen YC. Sleeve and sleeve-plus. Ann Laparosc Endosc Surg. 2017;2(24)

[2] World Health Organization. Obesity and overweight fact sheet [Internet]. 2020 [Updated 2020 April 1; cited 2020 October 8]. Available from: https://www.who.int/news-room/fact-sheets/detail/obesity-and-overweight

[3] Ohta M, Seki Y, Wong SK, Wang C, Huang CK, Aly A, et al. Bariatric/metabolic surgery in the Asia-Pacific region: APMBSS 2018 survey. Obes Surg. 2018 Oct 10;23(9):534-541.

[4] Agrawal, S. Obesity, bariatric and metabolic surgery: a practical guide. Switzerland: Springer; 2016 [cited 2020 Oct 12]. Available from: DOI:10.1007/978-3-319-04343-2

[5] International Federation for the Surgery of Obesity and Metabolic Discoders. 5th IFSO global registry report 2019. United Kingdom: Dendrite Clinical Systems Ltd; 2019. 100 p. Report No.: 5. Available from: https://www.ifso.com/pdf/5th-ifso-global-registry-report-september-2019.pdf

[6] Kremen AJ, Linner JH, Nelson CH. An experimental evaluation of the nutritional importance of proximal and distal small intestine. Ann Surg [Internet]. 1954 [cited 2020 Oct 10];140(3):439-48. Available from: DOI:10.1097_00000658-195409000-00018

[7] Lee WJ, Wang W. Bariatric surgery: Asia-Pacific perspective. Obes Surg [Internet]. 2005 [cited 2021 Jan 1];15:751-7. Available from: 10.1381/0960892054222614

[8] Griffen WO, Young VL, Stevenson CC. A prospective comparison of gastric and jejunoileal bypass procedures for morbid obesity. Ann Surg [Internet]. 1977 [cited 2020 Oct 13];186(4):500-9. Available from: DOI:10.1097/00000658-197710000-00012

[9] Milone L, Strong V, Gagner M. Laparoscopic sleeve gastrectomy is superior to endoscopic intragastric balloon as a first stage procedure for super-obese patients (BMI > or =50). Obesity surgery [Internet]. 2005 [cited 2020 Oct 12]:15(15):612-7. Available from: DOI:10.1381/0960892053923833

[10] Nguyen N, Hinojosa M, Smith B, Reavis K. Single laparoscopic incision transabdominal (SLIT) surgery – adjustable gastric banding: a novel minimally invasive surgical approach. Obes Surg [Internet]. 2008 [cited 2020 Oct 11] 18(12):1629-31. Available from: DOI:10.1007/s11695-008-9705-6

[11] Saber A, Elgamal M, Itawi E, Rao A. Single incision laparoscopic sleeve gastrectomy (SILS): a novel technique. Obes Surg [Internet]. 2008 [cited 2020 Oct 20];18(10):1338-42. Available from: DOI:10.1007/s11695-008-9646-0

[12] Huang CK, Houng JY, Chiang CJ, Chen YS, Lee HL. Single incision transumbilical laparoscopic roux-en-y gastric bypass: a first case report. Obes Surg [Internet]. 2009 [cited 2020 Oct 15];19(12):1711-15. Available from: DOI:10.1007/s11695-009-9900-0

[13] Huang CK, Lo CH, Houng, JY, Chen YS, Lee PH. Surgical results of single-incision transumbilical laparoscopic roux en y gastric bypass. Surg Obes Relat Dis [Internet]. 2010 [cited 2020 Oct 15];8(2): 201-7. Available from: DOI:10.1016/j.soard.2010.12.007

[14] Hess DS, Hess DW. Biliopancreatic diversion with a duodenal switch. Obes Surg [Internet]. 1998 [cited 2020 Oct 20];8(3):267-82. Available from: DOI:10.1381/096089298765554476

[15] Marceau P, Hould FS, Simard S, Lebel S, Bourque R-A, Potvin M, Biron S. Biliopancreatic diversion with duodenal switch. World J Surg [Internet]. 1998 [cited 2020 Oct 20]; 22(9):947-54. Available from: 10.1007/s002689900498

[16] Sánchez-Pernaute A, Rubio Herrera MA, Pérez-Aguirre E, García Pérez JC, Cabrerizo L, Díez Valladares L, et al. Proximal duodenal- ileal end-to-side bypass with sleeve gastrectomy: proposed technique. Obes Surg [Internet]. 2007 [cited 2020 Oct 21]; 17(12):1614-8. Available from: DOI: 10.1007/s11695-007-9287-8

[17] Santoro S, Castro LC, Velhote MC, Malzoni CE, Klajner S, Castro LP. Sleeve gastrectomy with transit bipartition: a potent intervention for metabolic syndrome and obesity. Ann Surg [Internet]. 2012 [cited 2020 Oct 16]; 256(1):104-110. Available from: DOI:10.1097/SLA.0b013e31825370c0

[18] Mui WL, Lee DW, Lam KK. Laparoscopic sleeve gastrectomy with loop bipartition: a novel metabolics operation in treating obese type II diabetes mellitus. Int J Surg Case Rep [Internet]. 2014 [cited 2020 Oct 16];5(2):56-8. Available from: DOI:10.1016/j.ijscr.2013.12.002

[19] Kasama K, Tagaya N, Kahenira E, Oshiro T, Seki Y, Kinouchi M, et al. Laparoscopic sleeve gastrectomy with duodenojejunal bypass: technique and preliminary results. Obes Surg [Internet]. 2009 [cited 2020 Oct 22]; 19(10):1341-5. Available from: DOI:10.1007/s11695-009-9873-z

[20] Huang CK, Goel R, Tai CM, Yen YC, Gohil V, Chen XY. Novel metabolic surgery for type II diabetes mellitus: loop duodenojejunal bypass with sleeve gastrectomy. Surg Laparosc Endosc Percutan Tech [Internet]. 2013 Dec [cited 2020 Oct 25];23(6):481-5. Available from: DOI:10.1097/SLE.0b013e3182950111

[21] Ugale S, Vennapusa A, Katakwar A, Ugale A. Laparoscopic bariatric surgery current trends and controversies. Ann Laparosc Endosc Surg [Internet]. 2017 [cited 2020 Nov 2];2(10):154. Available from: DOI:10.21037/ales.2017.07.02

[22] Alamo M, Sepúlveda Torres C, Zapata Perez L. Vertical isolated gastroplasty with gastro-enteral bypass: preliminary results. Obes Surg [Internet]. 2006 [cited 2020 Nov 1];16(3):353-8. Available from: DOI:10.1381/096089206776116534

[23] Leung WK, Wu MS, Kakugawa Y, Kim JJ, Yeoh KG, Goh KL. Asia Pacific Working Group on Gastric Cancer. Screening for gastric cancer in Asia: current evidence and practice. Lancet Oncol [Internet]. 2008 Mar [cited 2020 Oct 21]; 9(3):279-87. Available from: DOI:10.1016/S1470-2045(08)70072-X

[24] McCabe ME 4th, Dilly CK. New causes for the old problem of bile reflux gastritis. Clin Gastroenterol Hepatol [Internet]. 2018 [cited 2020 Oct 17]; 16(9):1389-92. Available from: DOI: 10.1016/j.cgh.2018.02.034

[25] Oh SY, Lee HJ, Yang HK. Pylorus-preserving gastrectomy for gastric cancer. J Gastric Cancer [Internet]. 2016 Jun [cited 2020 Oct 16];16(2),63-71. Available from: https://doi.org/10.5230/jgc.2016.16.2.63

[26] Lee WJ, Lee KT, Kasama K, Seiki Y, Ser KH, Chun SC, Chen JC, Lee YC. Laparoscopic single-anastomosis duodenal-jejunal bypass with sleeve gastrectomy (SASGDJB): short-term result and comparison with gastric bypass. Obes Surg [Internet]. 2014 Jan [cited 2020 Oct 15];24(1),109-13. Available from: DOI:10.1007/s11695-013-1067-z

[27] Peterli R, Steinert RE, Woelnerhanssen B, Peters T, Christoffel-Courtin C, Gass M, et al. Metabolic and hormonal changes after laparoscopic roux-en-y gastric bypass and sleeve gastrectomy: a randomized, prospective trial. Obes Surg [Internet]. 2012 May [cited 2020 Oct 25];22(5):740-8. Available from: DOI:10.1007/s11695-012-0622-3

[28] Nuack MA. Incretin based therapies for type 2 diabetes mellitus; properties functions and clinical implications. Am J Med [Internet]. 2011 [cited 2020 Nov 3]; 124(1 Suppl),S3-18. Available from: DOI: 10.1016/j.amjmed.2010.11.002

[29] Laferrere B. Bariatric surgery and obesity: influence on the incretins. Int J Obes Suppl [Internet]. 2016 Dec [cited 2020 Oct 18];6(Supple 1):S32-36. Available from: DOI: 10.1038/ijosup.2016.8

[30] Nauck MA, Meier JJ. Incretin hormones: their role in health and disease. Diabetes Obes Metab [Internet]. 2018 Feb [cited 2020 Oct 15];20(Suppl 1):5-21. Available from: DOI:10.1111/dom.13129

[31] Abdalla MM. Ghrelin – physiological functions and regulation. Eur Endocrinol [Internet]. 2015 Aug [cited 2020 Oct 15];11(2):90-5. Available from: DOI:10.17925/EE.2015.11.02.90

[32] Tsoli M, Chronaiou A, Kehagias I, Kalfarentzos F, Alexandrides TK. Hormone changes and diabetes resolution after biliopancreatic diversion and laparoscopic sleeve gastrectomy: a comparative prospective study. Surg Obes Relat Dis [Internet]. 2013 Sep-Oct [cited 2020 Oct 16];9(5):667-77. Available from: DOI:10.1016/j.soard.2012.12.006

[33] Korner J, Inabnet W, Febres G, Conwell IM, McMahon DJ, Salas R, et al. Prospective study of gut hormone and metabolic changes after adjustable gastric banding and roux-en-y gastric bypass. Int J Obes [Internet]. 2009 Jul [cited 2020 Oct 18];33(7):786-95. Available from: DOI:10.1038/ijo.2009.79

[34] National Institutes of Health (US). Gastrointestinal Surgery for Severe Obesity. National Institutes of Health Consens Statement Online. 1991 Mar 25-27 [cited 2020 Oct 10];9(1):1-20. Available from: https://consensus.nih.gov/1991/1991gisurgeryobesity084html.htm

[35] National Institute for Health and Care Excellence (UK). Obesity: identification, assessment and management clinical guideline (CG189). 2014 Nov 27 [cited 2020 Oct 10]. Available from: https://www.nice.org.uk/guidance/cg189/chapter/1-recommendations

[36] Rubino F, Nathan DM, Eckel R, Schauer PR, Alberti GM, Zimmet PZ, et al. Metabolic surgery in the treatment algorithm for type 2 diabetes: a joint statement by international diabetes organizations. Diabetes Care [Internet]. 2016 Jun [cited 2020 Oct 12];39(6):861-77. Available from: https://doi.org/10.2337/dc16-0236

[37] Hsu WC, Araneta MR, Kanaya AM, Chiang JL, Fujimoto W. BMI cut points to identify at-risk Asian Americans for type 2 diabetes screening. Diabetes Care [Internet]. 2015 Jan [cited 2020 Oct 10];38(1):150-8. Available from: DOI:10.2337/dc14-2391

[38] Molero J. A propensity score cohort study on the long-term safety and efficacy of sleeve gastrectomy in patients older than age 60. J Obes [Internet]. 2020 Jul 31 [cited 2020 Oct 13]: 8783260. DOI: 10.1155/2020/8783260

[39] Huang CK, Garg A, Kuao HC, Chang PC, Hsin MC. Bariatric surgery in old age: a comparative study of laparoscopic roux-en-y gastric bypass and sleeve gastrectomy in an Asia centre of excellence. J Biomed Res [Internet]. 2015 Apr [cited 2020 Oct

13];29(2):118-24. Available from: DOI:10.7555/JBR.29.20140108.

[40] Abbas M, Cumella L, Zhang Y, Choi J, Vemulapalli P, Melvin WS, et al. Outcomes of laparoscopic sleeve gastrectomy and roux-en-y gastric bypass in patients older than 60. Obes Surg [Internet]. 2015 Dec [cited 2020 Oct 16];25(12):2251-6. Available from: DOI: 10.1007/s11695-015-1712-9

[41] Leivonen MK, Juuti A, Jaser N, Mustonen H. Laparoscopic sleeve gastrectomy in patients over 59 years: early recovery and 12-month follow-up. Obes Surg [Internet]. 2011 [cited 2020 Oct 16];21(8):1180-7. Available from: https://doi.org/10.1007/s11695-011-0454-6

[42] Miller-Matero LR, Bryce K, Saulino CK, Dykhuis K, Genaw J, Carlin A. Problematic eating behaviors predict outcomes after bariatric surgery. Obes Surg [Internet]. 2018 Jul [cited 2020 Oct 17];28(7):1910-5. Available from: https://doi.org/10.1007/s11695-018-3124-0

[43] Livhits M, Mercado C, Yermilov I, Parikh J, Dutson E, Mehran A, et al. Preoperative predictors of weight loss following bariatric surgery: systematic review. Obes Surg [Internet]. 2012 Jan [cited 2020 Oct 19];22(1):70-89. Available from: DOI: 10.1007/s11695-011-0472-4

[44] Brunicardi FC. Schwartz' Principles of Surgery. 10th ed. United States of America: McGraw-Hill Education. 2015

[45] Huang CK, Mahendra R, Hsin MC, Chang PC. Novel metabolic surgery: first Asia series and short-term results of laparoscopic proximal jejunal bypass with sleeve gastrectomy. Ann Laparosc Endosc Surg [Internet]. 2016 Dec [cited 2020 Oct 17];1(7):37. Available from: DOI:10.21037/ales.2016.10.05.

[46] Gu L, Huang X, Li S, Mao D, Shen Z,Khadaroo PA, et al. A meta-analysis of the medium- and long-term effects of laparoscopic sleeve gastrectomy and laparoscopic roux-en-y gastric bypass. BMC Surg [Internet]. 2020 Feb [cited 2020 Oct 21];20(1):30. Available from: DOI:10.1186/s12893-020-00695-x

[47] Hu Z, Sun J, Li R Wang Z, Ding H, Zhu T, et al. A comprehensive comparison of LRYGB and LSG in obese patients including the effects on QoL, co-morbidities, weight loss, and complications: a systematic review and meta-analysis. Obes Surg [Internet]. 2020 Mar [cited 2020 Nov 3];30(3):819-27. Available from: DOI: 10.1007/s11695-019-04306-4

[48] Switzer NJ, Prasad S, Debru E, Church N, Mitchell P, Gill R. Sleeve gastrectomy and type 2 diabetes mellitus: a systematic review of long-term outcomes. Obes Surg [Internet]. 2016 July [cited 2020 Oct 22]; 26(7):1616-21. Available from: DOI:10.1007/s11695-016-2188-y

[49] Ferzli GS, Dominique E, Ciaglia M, Bluth MH, Gonzalez A, Fingerhut A. Clinical improvement after duodenojejunal bypass for nonobese type 2 diabetes despite minimal improvement in glycemic homeostasis. World J Surg [Internet]. 2009 [cited 2020 Oct 22];33(5):972-9. Available from: DOI: 10.1007/s00268-009-9968-7

[50] Paik KY, Kim W, Song KH, Kwon HS, Kim MK, Kim E. The preliminary clinical experience with laparoscopic duodenojejunal bypass for treatment of type 2 diabetes mellitus in non-morbidly obese patients: the 1-year result in a single institute. Surg Endosc [Internet]. 2012 [cited 2020 Oct 23]; 26(11):3287-92. Available from: DOI: 10.1007/s00464-012-2341-1

[51] Raj P, Kumaravel R, Chandramaliteeswaran C, Rajpandian S, Palanivelu C. Is laparoscopic duodenojejunal bypass with sleeve an

effective alternative to roux en y gastric bypass in morbidly obese patients: preliminary results of a randomized trial. Obes Surg [Internet]. 2012 [cited 2020 Oct 22];22(3):422-6. Available from: DOI:10.1007/s11695-011-0507-x

[52] Lee WJ, Almulaifi AM, Tsou JJ, Ser KH, Lee YC, Chen SC. Duodenal–jejunal bypass with sleeve gastrectomy versus the sleeve gastrectomy procedure alone: the role of duodenal exclusion. Surg Obes Relat Dis [Internet]. 2015 July-August [cited 2020 Oct 24];11(4):765-70. Available from: DOI: 10.1016/j.soard.2014.12.017

[53] Seki Y, Kasama K, Umezawa A, Kurokawa Y. Laparoscopic sleeve gastrectomy with duodenojejunal bypass for type 2 diabetes mellitus. Obes Surg [Internet]. 2016 September [cited 2020 Oct 21];26(9),2035-44. Available from: DOI:10.1007/s11695-016-2057-8

[54] Seki Y, Kasama K, Haruta H, Watanabe H, Yokoyama R, Porciuncula JP, et al. Five-year-results of laparoscopic sleeve gastrectomy with duodenojejunal bypass for weight loss and type 2 diabetes mellitus. Obes Surg [Internet]. 2017 Mar [cited 2020 Oct 22]; 27(3):795-801. Available from: DOI: 10.1007/s11695-016-2372-0

[55] Huang CK, Tai CM, Chang PC, Malapan K, Tsai CC, Yolsuriyanwong K. Loop duodenojejunal bypass with sleeve gastrectomy: comparative study with roux-en-y gastric bypass in type 2 diabetic patients with a BMI <35 kg/m2, first year results. Obes Surg [Internet]. 2016 October [cited 2020 Oct 23]; 26(10): 2291-3201. Available from: DOI:10.1007/s11695-016-2118-z

[56] Hanipah ZN, Hsin MC, Liu CC, Huang CK. Laparoscopic loop duodenaljejunal bypass with sleeve gastrectomy in type 2 diabetic patients. Surg Obes Relat Dis [Internet]. 2019 May [cited 2020 Nov 3];15(5):696-702. Available from: DOI:10.1016/j.soard.2019.01.016

[57] Sepulveda M, Alamo M, Lynch R, Castillo G, Preiss Y, Prat X. Comparison of long-term weight loss between sleeve gastrectomy and sleeve gastrectomy with jejunal bypass. Surg Obes Relat Dis [Internet]. 2017 Oct [cited 2020 Nov 1]; 13(10):S58. Available from: https://doi.org/10.1016/j.soard.2017.09.128

[58] Alamo M, Sepulveda M, Astorga C, Lagos J, Penaloza L, Montes B. Sleeve gastrectomy with jejunal bypass: excess weight loss after 10 years of follow up. In: proceedings of the 19th World Congress of the International Federation for the Surgery of Obesity (IFSO'14). Obes Surg [Internet]. 2015 Aug 26-30 [cited 2020 Oct 31];24:1178-9.

[59] Alamo M, Sepulveda M, Gellona J, Herrera M, Astorga C, Manterola C. Sleeve gastrectomy for the treatment of type 2 diabetes mellitus in patients with body mass index of <35 kg/m2: a cohort study. Obes Surg [Internet]. 2012 [cited 2020 Nov 2];22(7):1097-103. Available from: DOI: 10.1007/s11695-012-0652-x

[60] Sepulveda M, Alamo M, Preiss Y, Valderas J. Metabolic surgery comparing sleeve gastrectomy with jejunal bypass and roux-en-y gastric bypass in type 2 diabetic patients after 3 years. Obes Surg [Internet]. 2018 Nov [cited 2020 Oct 23];28(11):3466-73. Available from: DOI:10.1007/s11695-018-3402-x

[61] Lin S, Guan W, Yang N, Zang Y, Liu R, Liang H. Short-term outcomes of sleeve gastrectomy plus jejunojejunal bypas: a retrospective comparative study with sleeve gastrectomy and roux-en-y gastric bypass in chinese patients with BMI >35kg/m2. Obes Surg [Internet]. 2019 Apr [cited 2020 Nov 3];29(4):1352-9. Available from: D OI:10.1007/s11695-018-03688-1

[62] Masoomi H, Nguyen NT, Stamos MJ, Smith BR. Overview of

outcomes of laparoscopic and open roux-en-y gastric bypass in the United States. Surg Technol Int [Internet]. 2012 Dec [cited 2020 Nov3];22: 72-6. Available from: DOI: https://pubmed.ncbi.nlm.nih.gov/23065805/

[63] Stenberg E, Szabo E, Agren G, Näslund E, Boman L, Bylund A, et al. Early complications after laparoscopic gastric bypass surgery: results from the Scandinavian Obesity Surgery Registry. Ann Surg [Internet]. 2014 [cited 2020 Nov 4];260(6),1040-1047. https://doi.org/10.1097/SLA.0000000000000004

[64] Kehagias I, Karamanakos SN, Argentou M, Kalfarentzos F. Randomized clinical trial of laparoscopic roux-en-y gastric bypass versus laparoscopic sleeve gastrectomy for the management of patients with BMI < 50 kg/m2. Obes Surg [Internet]. 2011 [cited 2020 Oct 28];21(11):1650-6. Available from: https://doi.org/10.1007/s11695-011-0479-x

[65] Lager CJ, Esfandiari NH, Subauste AR, et al. Roux-en-y gastric bypass vs. sleeve gastrectomy: balancing the risks of surgery with the benefits of weight loss. Obes Surg [Internet]. 2017 [cited 2020 Nov 2];27(1):154-61. Available from: DOI:10.1007/s11695-016-2265-2

[66] Salminen P, Helmiö M, Ovaska J, et al. Effect of laparoscopic sleeve gastrectomy vs. laparoscopic roux-en-y gastric bypass on weight loss at 5 years among patients with morbid obesity: the SLEEVEPASS randomized clinical trial. *JAMA [Internet]*. 2018 [cited 2020 Nov 5];319(3),241-54. Available from: DOI:10.1001/jama.2017.20313

[67] Dick A, Byrne TK, Baker M, Budak A, Morgan K. Gastrointestinal bleeding after gastric bypass surgery: nuisance or catastrophe?. Surg Obes Relat Dis [Internet]. 2010 [cited 2020 Oct 28];6(6):643-7. Available from: https://doi.org/10.1016/j.soard.2010.07.016

[68] Frezza EE, Reddy S, Gee LL, Wachtel MS. Complications after sleeve gastrectomy for morbid obesity. Obes Surg [Internet]. 2009 [cited 2020 Oct 21];19(6):684-7. Available from: https://doi.org/10.1007/s11695-008-9677-6

[69] Gagner M, Kemmeter P. Comparison of laparoscopic sleeve gastrectomy leak rates in five staple-line reinforcement options: a systematic review. Surg Endosc [Internet]. 2020 [cited 2020 Nov 3]; 34(1): 396-407. Available from: https://doi.org/10.1007/s00464-019-06782-2

[70] Alizadeh RF, Li S, Inaba C, Penalosa P, Hinojosa MW, Smith BR, Stamos MJ, Nguyen NT. Risk factors for gastrointestinal leak after bariatric surgery: MBASQIP analysis. J Am Coll Surg [Internet]. 2018 [cited 2020 Oct 28];227(1):135-41. Available from: https://doi.org/10.1016/j.jamcollsurg.2018.03.030

[71] Burgos AM, Braghetto I, Csendes A, Maluenda F, Korn O, Yarmuch J, et al. Gastric leak after laparoscopic-sleeve gastrectomy for obesity. Obes Surg [Internet]. 2009 [cited 2020 Oct 28]; 19(12):1672-7. Available from: https://doi.org/10.1007/s11695-009-9884-9

[72] Brethauer S, Schauer P, Schirmer B. Minimally invasive bariatric surgery. 2nd ed. New York: Springer Science+Business Media. 2015. Available from: DOI:10.1007/978-1-4939-1637-5

[73] Yeung K, Penney N, Ashrafian L, Darzi A, Ashrafian H. Does sleeve gastrectomy expose the distal esophagus to severe reflux?: a systematic review and meta-analysis. Ann Surg [Internet]. 2020 [cited 2020 Nov 3];271(2):257-65. Available from: DOI:10.1097/SLA.0000000000003275

[74] Soricelli E, Iossa A, Casella G, Abbatini F, Calì B, Basso N. Sleeve gastrectomy and crural repair in obese patients with gastroesophageal reflux disease and/or hiatal hernia. Surg

Obes Relat Dis [Internet]. 2013 [cited 2020 Nov 5];9(3):356-61. Available from: https://doi.org/10.1016/j.soard.2012.06.003

[75] Parikh A, Alley JB, Peterson RM, Harnisch MC, Pfluke JM, Tapper DM, et al. Management options for symptomatic stenosis after laparoscopic vertical sleeve gastrectomy in the morbidly obese. Surg Endosc [Internet]. 2012 [cited 2020 Nov 4];26(3):738-46. Available from: https://doi.org/10.1007/s00464-011-1945-1

[76] Vilallonga R, Himpens J, van de Vrande S. Laparoscopic management of persistent strictures after laparoscopic sleeve gastrectomy. Obes Surg [Internet]. 2013 [cited 2020 Oct 18];23(10):1655-61. Available from: https://doi.org/10.1007/s11695-013-0993-0

[77] Chiu CC, Lee WJ, Wang W, Wei PL, Huang MT. Prevention of trocar wound hernia in laparoscopic bariatric operations. Obes Surg [Internet] 2006 [cited 2020 Nov 3];16(7):913-8. Available from: DOI: 10.1381/096089206777822269

[78] Lin S, Yang N, Guan W, Liang W. Can Chinese t2d patients with BMI 20-32.5 kg/m^2 benefit from loop duodenojejunal bypass with sleeve gastrectomy? Surg Obes Relat Dis [Internet]. 2019 [cited 2020 Nov 3];15(9);1513-9. Available from: DOI:10.1016/j.soard.2019.03.027

[79] Huang CK, Katakwar A. Sleeve-plus procedures: need of time. Surg Today [Internet]. 2019 Oct 10 [cited 2020 Nov 5]; 50(4):419-22. Available from: DOI: 10.1007/s00595-019-01895-6

Chapter 8

Weight Regain and Insufficient Weight Loss after Bariatric Surgery: A Call for Action

Wahiba Elhag and Walid El Ansari

Abstract

Despite successful weight loss after bariatric surgery (BS), weight regain (WR) may occur on long term following most bariatric procedures, with 20–30% of patients either failing to reach their target weight goals or failing to maintain the achieved weight loss. Significant WR has important health consequences, including the reversal of the improved obesity-related comorbidities and psychological function leading to decreased quality of life. Given the challenges faced by these patients, there is a need for multidisciplinary approaches to deal with WR. This chapter addresses the issue of WR among bariatric patients. It starts with the various definitions of insufficient weight loss and WR and the prevalence of weight regain by type of bariatric procedure. The chapter then explores the underlying causes as well as the predictors of WR. It will also outline the behavioral and psychotherapeutic, dietary and exercise strategies employed in the prevention of post-surgery WR. The chapter will then highlight the non-surgical and surgical approaches used in the management of WR. The chapter will conclude with a summary of the findings emphasizing that WR is complex and multifactorial, requiring multidisciplinary and multimodal dietary, behavioral, pharmacological, and surgical management strategies tailored to meet the individual needs of each patient.

Keywords: bariatric surgery, weight regain, insufficient weight loss, causes, predictors, management

1. Introduction

Bariatric surgery (BS) can achieve weight loss (WL), treat obesity-related metabolic disease and enhance the metabolic status by improving hypertension, type 2 diabetes mellitus (T2DM) and lipid profile, thereby decreasing the cardiovascular risk [1, 2]. Despite effective WL after BS, some patients do not achieve their target weight goals, and others regain a significant portion of their weight at long-term follow-up. Weight regain (WR) has a range of undesirable medical and psychological impacts [3, 4].

WR might occur after common BS procedures e.g. gastric bypass, adjustable gastric banding (LAGB), and sleeve gastrectomy (LSG), to different extents and at variable interval times [5]. The causes for WR are multifactorial, including patient- and procedure-specific factors [6, 7]. Interestingly, WR might occur despite the patients' stated adherence to advised behavioral measures and absence of surgical anatomic causes. This suggests that various pre or post-operative demographic, physiologic or metabolic features could play a role. Given the complexity of the factors involved in WR, multimodal management strategies tailored to meet the individual needs of patients are essential.

2. Definitions of insufficient weight loss and weight regain

There is a distinction between two types of WL failure post BS: insufficient WL (IWL); and WR. The grouping of these two categories together should be discouraged. IWL is defined as excess weight loss (EWL%) of <50% at 18 months after BS [8], while WR is defined as regain of weight that occurs after achievement of an initial successful weight loss (defined as EWL% > 50%).

A range of definitions describe WR post BS [9, 10]. The lack of standard definition, consensus statements and guidelines leads to poor reporting and understanding of the significance of WR [3, 8, 10]. Moreover, clearer definitions will help to recognize when intervention is required and guide the intervention [8]. Available definitions include: regaining weight reaching a body mass index (BMI) >35 after successful WL [11]; an increase in BMI of $\geq$5 kg/m^2 above the nadir weight [12]; > 25% EWL% regain from nadir [13, 14]; increase in weight of >10 kg from nadir [15, 16]; any WR [17]; any WR after type 2 diabetes mellitus (T2DM) remission [18]; or an increase of >15% of total body weight from nadir [19, 20]. The most common definition, an increase of $\geq$10 kg of nadir weight [15, 21], does little to define the clinical significance of the amount of WR in the affected individual. Therefore, a WR definition needs to be meaningful rather than arbitrary. It is important to note that multiple definitions affect the reporting of the prevalence of WR, and considerably change the reported outcomes. For instance, applying 6 different WR definitions to 55 patients 5 years after LSG led to WR rates ranging from 9–91% [10]. Similarly, the use of 5 continuous and 8 dichotomous measures among 1406 Roux en Y gastric bypass (RYGB) patients followed up for 5 years resulted in WR rates ranging from 44–87% [9]; and others reported rates between 16–37% WR 5 years post LAGB, LSG, and RYGB [19]. Therefore, more research is needed to define WR after BS in order to standardize its measurement.

3. Prevalence of WR and IWL after bariatric procedures

WR following BS varies by the type of BS performed, whether restrictive or malabsorptive as outlined below.

3.1 Laparoscopic gastric band (LAGB)

A large prospective multicenter study in Sweden found that 10 years post LAGB, patients regained 38% of the maximal weight they lost post surgery [1]. Likewise, research at 10 US hospitals that assessed weight trajectories among 2348 participants including 610 LAGB patients reported 1.4% WR 3 to 7 years after surgery [22] (**Table 1**).

3.2 Laparoscopic sleeve gastrectomy (LSG)

A systematic review of 21 studies reported WR rates post LSG ranging from 5.7% at 2 years to 76% over variable follow-up periods from (2 to 6 years) [3].

Type of BS	Prevalence of WR
LAGB	1.4% between years 3 and 7 years [22] 38% at 10 years [1]
LSG	5.7% at 2 years [3] 39.5% at 5 years [23] 76% over variable follow-up periods ranging from 2 to 6 years [3]
RYGB	17.1% at 2 years [24] 22.5% at 3 years [9] 14.6%–26.8% at 5 years [9, 25] 3.9% between 3 and 7 years [22]

LAGB: Laparoscopic gastric band; LSG: Laparoscopic sleeve gastrectomy; RYGB: Roux en Y gastric bypass.

Table 1.
Prevalence of WR by type of BS.

Other studies found that WR started three years after LSG [23]. At 5 years, WR (>10 kg) was observed in 39.5% of patients, where the EWL% decreased from 84.8% at one year to 57.3% after 5 years [23].

3.3 Roux en Y gastric bypass (RYGB)

Research among 1426 patients found that at 2 years, 17.1% regained >15% of their 1-year post-operative weight [24]. Others reported a 22.5% WR at 3 years and 26.8% at 5 years [9]. The Longitudinal Assessment of Bariatric Surgery (LABS) study observed 3.9% WR between 3 and 7 years post RYGB [22]. Others found that among 2965 patients, WR was 14.6% at 5 years post-surgery [25].

4. Causes of WR

Causes of WR following BS are multifactorial, and can be categorized into patient- and surgical-specific causes. The former includes hormonal causes and maladaptive lifestyle behaviors (e.g. dietary non-compliance and physical inactivity) [3, 7]. Other factors include the lack of follow-up support and mental health causes such as psychiatric conditions and maladaptive eating [3, 7]. Surgical-specific factors include e.g., enlargement of the gastric pouch or gastro-gastric fistula. Recognizing such underling etiologies is key to develop appropriate management strategies [26]. **Figure 1** depicts the causes of WR.

4.1 Hormonal

Weight reduction following BS may be dependent to some extent on the 'normalization' of hormonal inputs. Furthermore, patients who fail to achieve WL post-BS or experience WR may have persistent hormonal 'imbalances' (e.g. high ghrelin, low peptide YY) which need to be addressed in order to accomplish WL.

Ghrelin is a hormone that is important in regulating food intake and energy balance. BS has a positive effect on ghrelin, where a significant decrease in both fasting and post prandial ghrelin is observed early after BS leading to decreased appetite and food intake [27]. However, research have found that among RYGB patients, subjects with WR had significantly higher pre and postoperative ghrelin levels compared to those who maintained or lost weight (722 ± 29 vs. 540 ± 156 pg/ml) [28]. Similarly, patients with WR 5 years post LSG had higher plasma ghrelin levels than their level at 1 year post surgery [16].

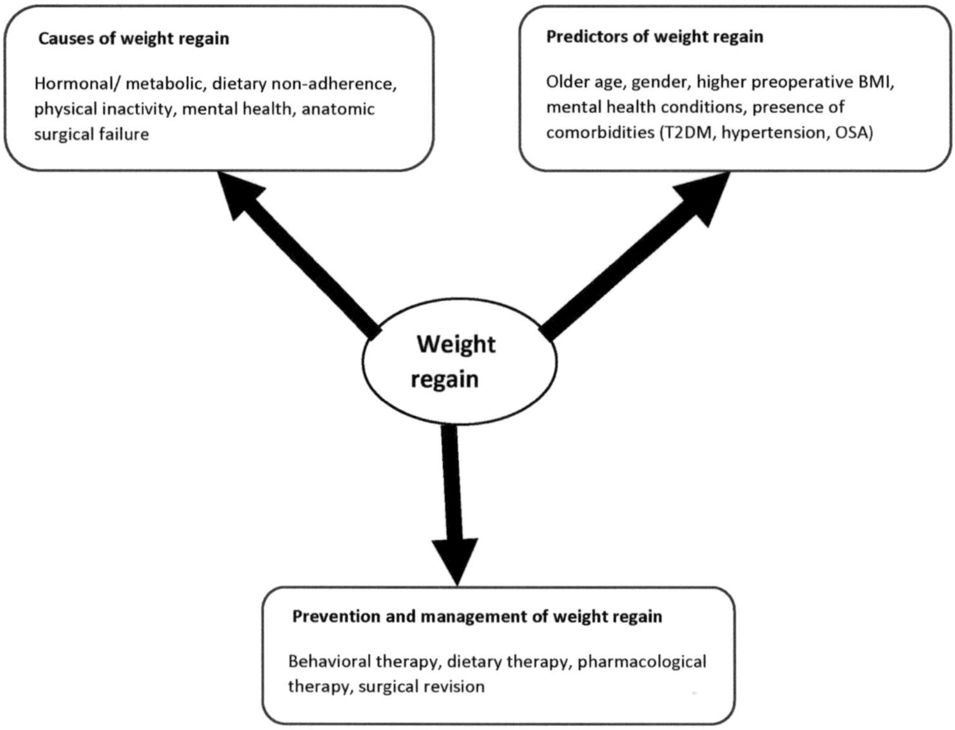

Figure 1.
Summary of the causes, predictors and prevention and management strategies of weight regain.

Peptide YY (PYY) is a 36 amino acid hormone that is released by the L-cells of the gastrointestinal tract after food intake to suppress appetite. Likewise, Glucagon-like protein-1 (GLP-1) is released after meals by L cells in the small intestine to stimulate insulin secretion, inhibit glucagon release, and delay gastric emptying [29]. Both these anorexigenic hormones display enhanced nutrient-stimulated secretion after BS, more so after RYGB than LSG [29]. However, the level of theses hormones was noticed to be lower in patients with WR. For instance, meal-stimulated gastric inhibitory polypeptide and glucagon-like peptide-1 (GLP-1) levels at 30 min were lower in 10 patients who had WR compared with 14 patients who successfully maintained WL post RYGB [30]. Whilst hormonal adaptation as a biological response to non-surgical WL has been examined [31], its influence on WR post BS is less documented in humans. For example, rodent studies showed that postsurgical WR was associated with failure to maintain elevated plasma PYY concentrations [32].

4.2 Nutritional non-adherence

Immediately following BS, caloric intake is reduced due to a smaller gastric capacity, diminished hunger, and increased satiety brought about by the anatomical and metabolic changes. Nevertheless, for some patients, caloric intake gradually increases over time which contributes to postoperative WR. In the Swedish Obesity Study, mean daily intakes of 2900, 1500, 1700,1800, 1900, and 2000 kcal/day were observed at baseline, 6 months, 12 months, 2 years, 3 years, and 4–10 years postsurgery respectively [1]. Such increase in food intake often begins in the second post-operative year, likely causing WR [1]. In addition, dietary non-adherence and the consumption of high-calorie foods and beverages contribute to the higher caloric intake leading to WR. A postoperative behavioral survey of 203 patients observed positive correlations between the magnitude of WR and evening or night consumption of large quantities of food, eating large amounts of high-fat foods, and eating out more frequently [33]. Equally, among 289 RYGB patients, 23% demonstrated dietary non-adherence and a continuation of pre-surgical eating patterns, leading to suboptimal weight loss and WR [34]. Such evidence substantiate the importance of diet quality and caloric intake as causative factors for WR after BS, and also highlight the importance of measuring and documenting the diet quality after BS [35].

Grazing behavior is the repeated episodes of consumption of smaller quantities of food over a long period of time accompanied by feelings of loss of control [36]. Those engaging in grazing nibbled continuously ≥2 days per week for a 6-month period, with an inability to stop or control their eating while nibbling [36]. Grazing contributes to poor weight outcomes post BS [37]. Although grazing and binge eating are similar as they involve subjective episodes of food consumption accompanied by a loss of control; however, grazing is physiologically more possible post BS than large binges. In 80% of patients with preoperative binge eating or grazing with loss of control, these behaviors returned 6 months post-surgery [36]. This suggests that preoperative binge eating may reemerge as postsurgical grazing in the context of a reduced stomach capacity [36].

Food indiscretion also contributed to WR. For instance, the follow up of 100 patients for 85 months after surgery revealed that poor dietary habits including consumption of excessive calories, snacks, sweets oils and fatty foods were statistically higher in WR patients [6]. This highlightes the importance of appropriate nutritional counselling for long-term weight maintenance. Lack of appropriate nutritional follow-up was also significantly associated with WR post BS [6]. For example, studies have found that among those with WR post-RYGB, 60% never maintained follow-up with appropriate nutritional consultants [38].

4.3 Physical Inactivity

Inadequate physical activity contributes to WR. Only 10–24% of BS patients met the guidelines regarding minimal physical activity for health promotion (i.e., ≥150 min/week or moderate-to-vigorous physical activity in bouts of ≥10 min) [39]. A meta-analysis of 14 studies and a literature review of 19 studies concluded that post-BS physical activity was significantly associated with greater WL [40]. Amongst 100 obese patients post-RYGB, those who performed physical activity had the lowest incidence of WR compared to those who were relatively inactive [6]. Barriers to exercise among bariatric patients such as health concerns, lack of proximity to a gym/park, or feeling self-conscious should be identified and addressed [40]. Such findings highlight the importance of measuring and documenting physical activity levels after BS [35].

Similarly, sedentary behavior, defined as 'any waking behavior performed while in a sitting or reclining posture that requires very low energy expenditure'. The represents a risk factor for WR Sedentary behavior is associated with increased risk of obesity and related comorbidities [40]. Research have found that severely obese BS candidates are at high risk for SB [41]. In this study they found that BS candidates spent about 30% of their sedentary time watching television, suggesting that this is an important cause of sedentary behavior and should be a target for patient counseling [41].

4.4 Mental health

Mental health status prior to surgery is linked to WL following BS. Therefore, pre-operative psychological evaluation is important. Psychological factors might interfere with successful WL by undermining motivation, diet and exercise compliance, and other health behaviors critical to maintaining WL [42]. Among

60 adults who underwent RYGB or LAGB, 40% and 33.4% had single or multiple psychiatric diagnoses respectively, 47.5% stopped losing weight after 1 year, and 29.5% regained weight [43]. Furthermore, patients with ≥2 psychiatric conditions were 6 times more likely to either stop losing weight or regain weight relative to those with no or single psychiatric diagnosis [43]. Evidence supports the association between post-operative depressive disorders and poorer WL; however, the directionality of the relationship remains unknown [44]. More research is required to assess the long-term associations and directionality of depression and weight loss post BS.

4.5 Maladaptive eating: Binge eating (BE) disorder

Maladaptive eating patterns after BS have impact on weight and psychological outcomes [45]. One of these abnormal eating patterns is BE disorder which is defined as 'the consumption of large quantities of food during a short amount of time without being in control of this behavior', and is strongly associated with psychological distress [26]. BE disorder predicts poorer weight outcomes post BS, resulting in smaller BMI reductions as well as more WR [46, 47]. Despite the physical limitations of BS on stomach capacity, BE is not always abolished and many of those who had BE before BS still had feelings of loss of control when eating even small amounts of food post BS [37, 47]. Following RYGB, patients who regained >10% of their EWL% had significantly higher frequencies of BE and loss of control [46], and these maladaptive eating behaviors were significantly correlated with greater WR [46]. Follow up of 96 patients post RYGB two to seven years after surgery showed that binge eaters increased their BMI by 5.3 kg/m^2 compared with 2.4 kg/m^2 increase in non-binge eaters [48]. Likewise, among LAGB patients, the prevalence of eating disorder increased from 26.3% to 38.0% over one year post surgery, an increase that correlated with poorer WL outcomes [37].

4.6 Anatomic surgical failure

Each type of BS has its own potential mechanism/s of surgical failure that can lead to WR as outlined below.

4.6.1 Laparoscopic gastric band

LAGB success is correlated with appropriate follow-up, as saline adjustment of the band is essential for proper restriction and WL. Therefore, it is important to assess patients with WR after LAGB for potential pouch distension. Pouch distension is managed conservatively by complete band deflation, low calorie diet, reinforcement of portion size, and follow-up contrast study in 4–6 weeks, with success in more than 70% of patients [49]. On the other hand, premature removal of LAGB also causes WR. Studies have found that only 12% of patients with early band removal maintained their current weight [50]. Long term, LAGB removal rate is high, reaching 12% [51]. Moreover, after 14 years, the reoperation rate was as high as 30.5% with an average reoperation rate of 2.2% for every year of follow-up [51]. The main reason for LAGB removal was intolerance secondary to increased reflux type symptoms [52].

4.6.2 Laparoscopic sleeve gastrectomy

There are surgical causes of WR post LSG. The gastric sleeve may dilate over time leading to reduced restrictive effect and increase in gastric capacity, both associated with reduced satiety response and increased food intake resulting in WR [23]. For instance, among the 15.7% patients who had WR, CT scan volumetry showed that the mean gastric volume increased from 120 mL early after surgery to a mean of 240 mL at 3 years and to 524 mL at 5 years follow-up [23]. Several theories have been proposed as to the relationship of increased gastric volume and WR. One theory is that the physiologic dilation of the remnant stomach over time and the size of the gastric sleeve are linearly correlated with post-operative BMI [53, 54]. Another theory is the incomplete removal of the gastric fundus [55, 56], where in many cases, the dissection over the fundus, especially on the posterior aspect, may be difficult and technically demanding, notably in patients with the extreme obesity. Therefore, the success of LSG depends on the surgeon's learning curve [55].

4.6.3 Roux-en-Y gastric bypass

RYGB produces WL through restriction of intake and malabsorption. In assessing WR post-RYGB, anatomical abnormalities are proposed to play a role. Dilatation of the gastric pouch or gastrojejunostomy (GJ) stoma outlet have been associated with loss of satiety with subsequent increase in food intake and WR [57, 58]. Among 205 RYGB patients who had upper endoscopy as workup for WR, dilation of the GJ was identified in 58.9%, enlarged gastric pouch in 28.8%, and both abnormalities in 12.3% of patients [57]. Multivariate analysis found that stoma diameter (>2 cm) was independently associated with WR [58], where among 28 patients following RYGB, WR was associated with dilated gastric stoma [59]. In this group, successful reduction in anastomotic size (<12 mm) with a sclerotic agent resulted in a mean 26-kg WL at 18 months [59].

Another anatomic change that reduces RYGB'S effectiveness is gastro-gastric fistula, an abnormal communication between the gastric pouch and the excluded stomach. This is thought to develop as a result of the breakdown of the surgical staple line. Although gastro-gastric fistulas are uncommon, with a 1.5–6% incidence rate [60]. Gastro-gastric fistulas have potentially significant effects as a complication after RYGB [60] as they may diminish the restrictive and malabsorptive components of RYGB leading WR [61].

5. Predictors of WR post BS

Knowledge of the preoperative predictors of WR post-BS can assist in identifying patients at risk for WR. The bariatric team can then offer such patients appropriate resources and counseling. **Figure 1** depicts the predictors of WR.

5.1 Age

Age seems to be a predictor of WR, however, findings are inconsistent. Some smaller studies identified older age as a potential preoperative predictor of WR [62, 63]. Among 227 patients who underwent RYGB, older age (>60 years) predicted inadequate EWL% at 12 months [62]. While others found that younger individuals were more likely to have WR after RYGB [24].

5.2 Gender

Among post RYGB patients, male sex was associated with a worse weight trajectory [22] and suboptimal WL at 1 year after surgery [64]. Others found no effect of gender on weight loss outcomes [62].

5.3 Duration since surgery

Longer duration after BS predicted WR [24]. One study reported significant longer time since RYGB surgery in patients with WR (6 years) compared with patients who sustained their weight loss (3.3 years) [24]. Longer durations after surgery are probably associated with resolution of food intolerances, return to preoperative eating and other lifestyle patterns, anatomic surgical failure, or poor attendance of postoperative appointments [7, 65].

5.4 Preoperative BMI

Greater preoperative BMI was significantly associated with IWL [64]. A meta-analysis found that preoperative BMI and super-obesity were negatively associated with WL, where super-obese patients had 10.1 EWL% decrease [66]. Others observed that at 12 months post RYGB or LAGB, patients with baseline BMI $\geq$ 50 kg/m^2 were more likely to have significant WR, but those with BMI < 50 kg/m^2 were likely to continue losing weight [67]. Similarly, 80–100% of LSG patients with pre-surgery BMI > 40 kg/m^2 had WR to BMI > 30 kg/m^2 two years years after surgery; but only 3.6–38% of patients with lower pre-operative BMI (32.1–39.9 kg/m^2) had BMI > 30 kg/m^2 during the same time period [68].

5.5 Mental health

A presurgical BE disorder diagnosis predicted higher BMI. For example, studies found that among post-RYGB patients with 28.1 months mean follow-up, 79% reported WR and 15% regained $\geq$15% of their total weight loss [65]. The independent predictors of significant WR were lack of control of food urges (odds ratio, OR = 5.1), alcohol/drug use (OR = 12.74), lowest self-reported well-being scores (OR = 21.5), and lack of follow-up visits [65].

5.6 Presence of Comorbidities

Presence of T2DM predicts WR [22, 62, 63]. An assessment of 2348 bariatric participants in the Longitudinal Assessment of Bariatric Surgery (LABS) Study found that low HDL cholesterol and hypertension were also associated with an inferior weight trajectory [22].

6. Implications of weight regain

WR has important health consequences including recurrence of obesity related co-morbidities such as T2DM and deterioration in quality of life (QoL), thus contributing to socioeconomic and direct health care costs. This range of implications of WR is highlighted below.

6.1 Relapse of comorbidities

WR following BS is associated with and significantly predicted relapse of T2DM [12, 70]. At 10 year follow up, T2DM relapse was dependent on the extent of WR [70]. Patients with no WR had no relapse of their diabetes [70]. While, patients with mild regain (increase body weight > 5 kg from nadir) and severe regain (> 10 kg from nadir) had 5% and 17% relapse rates respectively [70]. Among 1406 RYGB patients with WR during the first year after reaching nadir weight, 25.8% and

46.2% of participants experienced progression of hyperlipidemia and hypertension respectively [9].

6.2 Quality of life

WR is significantly associated with deterioration in QoL [3, 9]. A study found that WR at 5 years after LSG was associated with a lower odds of satisfaction with surgery as measured by the Bariatric Analysis Reporting Outcome System (BAROS) score (incorporates weight loss, changes in medical conditions, health-related QoL, and reoperations) [3]. Others reported declines of physical and mental health–related QoL among 20.2% and 27.7% of patients with WR respectively [9]. Moreover, satisfaction with surgery also declined among 12.4% of patients with WR [9]. This decline was observed when the rate of WR was the highest, supporting a dose–response relationship (i.e., the less WR, the better) for physical health–related QoL [9].

7. Prevention of weight regain

Figure 1 summarizes the prevention strategies of WR. The foundation of prevention of WR after BS is aggressive behavioral interventions, similar to those utilized for medical weight management patients [33]. Behavioral modification components include commitment to regular structured physical activity, dietary control, nutritional optimization with substantive changes in eating practices and lifestyle habits [33, 71]. Other modulators include stress management, realistic goal setting, environmental control strategies, support systems, and cognitive restructuring [33, 71]. Close regular follow-up should start shortly after BS to reinforce nutritional and lifestyle instructions provided at discharge. Monitoring, education, and support should continue on the long term as the effectiveness of behavioral changes diminishes with time [33]. Self-monitoring with regular weight measurement, food records, and exercise diaries are essential tools for avoiding WR. These strategies increase patient's awareness of eating patterns, and allow the bariatric dietitian to identify high-risk areas, such as nutritional inadequacy, food intolerances, poor food choices, or food dislikes that compromise weight loss and nutritional status [72]. In-person dietary counseling by a registered dietitian has an important role in prevention of WR post BS [73]. Structured physical activity is vital for weight prevention. An RCT demonstrated that a 5-month supervised exercise program post LSG resulted in reduction total body weight (TBW) and waist circumference with an increase in EWL% compared with the control group [74]. Conversely, stopping of the exercise program led to weight regain, with increased fat mass and decreased EWL% [74].

8. Management of WR

Figure 1 illustrates the management strategies of WR. WR after BS is complex and multifactorial [7]. Hence, management requires a holistic strategy addressing patient- and surgery-related factors that might contribute to WR. Dietary patterns, psychological disorders and physical activity levels should all be reviewed, as diet (25.3%), physical activity (21%) and motivational issues (19.7%) were the most common reasons among patients with WR [75]. Patients seeking BS often present with a range of mental health issues including mood, anxiety, addiction and personality disorders [7, 26]. Diagnosis and management of these conditions may improve outcomes following BS. As the patient undergoes psychological, dietary and physical activity counselling, it is critical to address the hormonal causes, and any anatomic/post-surgical changes that cause WR. Baseline anatomic studies include esophagogastroduodenoscopy or an upper gastrointestinal contrast to evaluate the GI tract [76]. These modalities provide essential data about the gastric remnant size, size of the gastrojejunal anastomosis, presence of gastro-gastric fistula, and location/integrity of the bands. Available treatment options include behavior interventions, WL-approved medications, endoscopic interventions and revision surgery to counter some of the factors that resulted in WR.

8.1 Behavioral

Psychological and behavioral factors that have negative impact on long term WL outcomes include life stressors that derail weight maintenance and decreased adherence to the recommended postoperative diet. This is likely due to lack of psychological skills to engage in long term healthy eating behaviors. This is particualry important as the effects of surgery on appetite, hunger, and desire for food decrease. The aim is to address such challenges by behavioral therapy that is tailored to each patient's need [77, 78]. Many patients with WR are lost to follow up; therefore, open, non-judgmental strategies that support the actions that patients are doing well are critical to motivate and involve patients in management [76].

A 6-week intervention of cognitive and dialectical behavior therapies among 29 RYGB patients (93% female) with WR of 37% of the initial WL, found that treatment completers had 1.6 ± 2.38 kg mean weight decrease compared with non completers [79]. Moreover, patients who completed behavior therapy treatment had improvement in their depressive symptoms with decreased grazing patterns ($p \leq 0.01$), as well as subjective binge eating episodes ($p \leq 0.03$) compared to non-completers [79]. Likewise, a 10-week behavioral intervention of psychological skills to mitigate WR among 11 patients after BS was feasible, acceptable (72% retention), and with high satisfaction among completers (4.25 out of 5.00) [80]. WR was stopped or reversed, with a mean 3.58 ± 3.02% total body WL% [80]. Similarly, the use of acceptance-based strategies and online or phone intervention delivery modes to enhance outcomes and reach more patients showed feasibility, acceptability (70% retention), efficacy, high satisfaction score of (4.7 out of 5.0), and reversal of WR with a mean 5.1 ± 5.5% total WL% at 3-month follow-up [81].

8.2 Dietary

Structured dietary interventions assist patients to improve WL. A randomized controlled trial (RCT) assigned post RYGB patients into two groups: a structured dietary intervention incorporating portion-controlled foods vs. a control group [77]. Both groups received behavioral WL instructions (one 60-min session followed by 4 coaching telephone calls at monthly intervals). The intervention group had significantly reduced calorie intake at 4 months (−108 vs. 116 Kcal) and increased WL% at 4 and 6 months compared to the control group (−4.56% vs. −0.13%, −4.07% vs. −0.14%, respectively) [77]. Another 16-week RCT among women who regained ≥5% of their lowest post-RYGB weight found that whey protein supplementation promoted WL and fat mass loss, with preserved muscle mass, compared to controls who gained weight (0.42 kg) and fat mass [82].

8.3 Pharmacological

Prior to 2012, the only FDA-approved WL drugs were orlistat, a modestly effective pancreatic lipase inhibitor with some side effects and phentermine, a sympathomimetic appetite suppressant approved for short-term use [83]. Since 2012, 4 other WL medications were approved [83]: phentermine-topiramate, bupropion hydrochloride-naltrexone hydrochloride, liraglutide and lorcaserin hydrochloride (withdrawn due to cancer risk [84]). Since then, anti-obesity medications have been increasingly used to manage WR post-BS. In an assessment of anti-obesity medications for WR/IWL among 319 patients (258 RYGB, 61 LSG), 54% lost ≥5% of their TBW, with many high responders (30.3% of patients lost ≥10%, and 15% lost ≥15% of their TBW) [85]. Of the 14 FDA approved and off-label anti-obesity medications, only topiramate showed statistically significant WL, where patients were 1.9 times more likely to lose ≥10% of their TBW [85]. Regardless of the postoperative BMI, RYGB patients were significantly more likely to lose ≥5% of their TBW with anti-obesity medications [85]. Another study of individual and combined anti-obesity medications for WR post RYGB reported that patients who received medications achieved significantly more WL compared to those not using anti-obesity medications [86]. Additionally, there was slower overall WR in the anti-obesity medications group during long term (11 year) follow up [86].

Among young adults post RYGB and LSG, topiramate, phentermine, and/or metformin led to 54.1%, 34.3% and 22.9% of patients losing ≥5% ≥10% and ≥ 15%, of their weight respectively [87]. Again, RYGB had higher median WL% than LSG (−8.1% vs. −3.3%), with no differences whether the anti-obesity medications were started at weight plateau or after WR [87]. In another study, phentermine was compered to phentermine–topiramate combination among RYGB or LAGB patients with WR and WL plateau [88]. The study showed that phentermine and phentermine–topiramate patients lost 6.35 kg (12.8% EWL%) and 3.81 kg (12.9% EWL%) respectively at 90 days post treatment [88].

Liraglutide, a GLP-1 analogue with central and peripheral actions, inhibits glucagon secretion, increases insulin secretion, decreases the gastric emptying rate, and promotes satiety [89]. In a recently published study, among 117 patients with WR after RYGB, LAGB and LSG, the use of liraglutide 3 mg over a 7 month period resulted in statistically significant WL (-6.3 ± 7.7 kg, $P < .05$) compared to baseline regardless of the type of surgery [90]. Moreover, the decrease in weight remained significant even after one year of liraglutide use [30]. In this study, nausea was the most prevalent side effect (29.1% patients) [90].

8.4 Surgical

Revision of a previous BS are carried out due to surgical complications e.g., development of intractable marginal ulcer, gastro-gastric fistula, severe gastroesophageal reflux, and malnutrition [91]. Recently, revisional surgery is increasingly utilized for the management of WR [91, 92].

8.4.1 After failed LAGB

In patients with WR or IWL after gastric band, the surgical options include band removal and revisional BS. A retrospective study evaluated the outcomes of revision of LAGB for inadequate weight loss to LSG or single anastomosis duodenal switch and found that patients who underwent single anastomosis duodenal switch had significantly greater weight loss than LSG in the first year post surgery, with excess BMI loss percentage of 66.7% versus 51.5% [93]. In the same study, at >12 months post revision, both single anastomosis duodenal switch patients and LSG patients had adequate WL (79% for single anastomosis duodenal switch versus 67.8% for LSG) [93]. A systematic review compared the WL outcomes of conversion gastric band to LSG or RYGB and showed significant increase in EWL% in RYGB and patients than LSG patients at 12 and 24 months after revision [94].

However, no statistically significant change was observed in terms of EWL% after 3, 6, or 36 months post revision [94]. RYGB was also associated with a higher rate of complications, readmission and longer operative time [94].

8.4.2 After failed LSG

Several surgical interventions can be considered for failed LSG including conversion to RYGB, biliopancreatic diversion with duodenal switch (BPD/DS), one anastomosis gastric bypass (OAGB) or single anastomosis duodeno-ileal bypass with sleeve gastrectomy (SADI-S). Among 43 post LSG patients who had revisional surgery for IWL/WR (25 patients converted to BPD/DS, 18 to RYGB), the median EWL% after 34 months was significantly greater for BPD/DS compared to RYGB (59% vs. 23%) [14]. However, short-term complications and vitamin deficiencies were higher in BPD/DS compared with RYGB [14].

Conversions of LSG to OAGB or RYGB are also utilized to manage WR. At 12 months, mean total WL percentage was significantly higher in OAGB compared to RYGB (15.8 ± 7.8% vs. 10.3 ± 7.6%), with no differences in readmission and complications between the two procedures, suggesting that OAGB is safe after failed LSG [95]. However, long-term follow up including the risk of malnutrition is needed for a complete evaluation of OAGB as a revisional BS. Another study evaluating the conversion of LSG to four different gastric bypass procedures including proximal RYGB, type 2 distal RYGB, long biliopancreatic limb RYGB and OAGB showed that the long biliopancreatic limb RYGB and OAGB resulted in significant EWL% at 3 years (33.8% and 33.2% respectively). However, the effect lasted only for 2 years in the proximal RYGB (EWL% of 23.1%) [96].

SADI-S is a relatively new procedure utilized as an alternative to the current duodenal switch (DS) [97]. Outcomes of SADI-S as a revision after LSG showed 20.5% weight loss and 9.4 units BMI change two years post revision with 93.7% T2DM remission rate [98]. Additionally, there were no mortality or conversions to open surgery, and postoperative early and late complication rates were low (5.3% and 6.4% respectively) [98].

8.4.3 After failed RYGB

There seems no standardized approach to revisional surgery after failed RYGB. A systemic review of revision of RYGB for WR (799 studies, 866 patients) assessed 5 revisions: conversion to distal RYGB or BPD/DS, or revision of gastric pouch and anastomosis, revision with gastric band or endoluminal procedures [92]. At 3-years after revision, mean excess body mass index loss percentage for distal RYGB was 52.2%, for BPD/DS was 76%, for gastric pouch or anastomosis revision was 14%, for gastric banding revision was 47.3%, and for endoluminal procedures was 32.1% [92]. Amongst these revisions, gastric pouch or anastomosis revision had the lowest rates for major complications (3.5%), while DRYGB had the highest rate for major complications (11.9%) and mortality (0.6%) [92]. A recently published study showed promising short and long term results as regards to the conversion of RYGB to long biliopancreatic limb RYGB for the management of IWL, where patients achieved an additional excess EWL% ranging from 40.0% at 1 year to 45.3% at 6 years [99].

9. Conclusions

Although BS is an effective treatment for weight loss and comorbidities resolution, however WR may occur on the long term. The lack of a standard definition and consensus on what constitutes clinically significance WR leads to poor reporting of this entity which requires further research. The underlying factors that contribute to WR are multifactorial, including hormonal and surgical causes, nutritional noncompliance, physical inactivity, and mental health issues. Therefore, patients with significant WR following BS should undergo comprehensive evaluations to determine the underlying etiology. Management should focus on preventive and treatment strategies delivered in a multidisciplinary approach to include dietary intervention, behavioral counseling, lifestyle modifications, pharmacotherapy and, if indicated, surgical revision. Future research should focus to identify the etiological factors and effective intervention strategies.

Acknowledgements

The publication fees of this chapter was funded by a grant from Novo Nordisk.

Conflict of interest

None.

Abbreviations

BMI	body mass index
BPD/DS	laparoscopic biliopancreatic diversion with duodenal switch
BS	Bariatric surgery
EWL	excess weight loss
FDA	food and drug administration
GI	gastrointestinal
GLP-1	polypeptide and glucagon-like peptide-1
IWL	insufficient weight loss
LAGB	Laparoscopic gastric band
LSG	Laparoscopic sleeve gastrectomy
OAGB	one anastomosis gastric bypass
QoL	quality of life
RCT	randomized controlled trial
RYGB	Roux en Y gastric bypass
SADI-S	single anastomosis duodeno-ileal bypass with sleeve gastrectomy
T2DM	type 2 diabetes mellitus
TBW	total body weight
WL	weight loss
WR	weight regain

Author details

Wahiba Elhag[1] and Walid El Ansari[2,3,4]*

1 Department of Bariatric Surgery/Bariatric Medicine, Hamad General Hospital, 3050 Doha, Qatar

2 Department of Surgery, Hamad General Hospital, 3050 Doha, Qatar

3 College of Medicine, Qatar University, Doha, Qatar

4 Schools of Health and Education, University of Skovde, Skövde, Sweden

*Address all correspondence to: welansari9@gmail.com

References

[1] Sjöström L, Lindroos A-K, Peltonen M, et al. Lifestyle, diabetes, and cardiovascular risk factors 10 years after bariatric surgery. The New England Journal of Medicine. 2004;**351**:2683-2693

[2] Cho J-M, Kim HJ, Lo Menzo E, Park S, Szomstein S, Rosenthal RJ. Effect of sleeve gastrectomy on type 2 diabetes as an alternative treatment modality to Roux-en-Y gastric bypass: systemic review and meta-analysis. Surg Obes Relat Dis Off J Am Soc Bariatr Surg. 2015;**11**:1273-1280

[3] Lauti M, Kularatna M, Hill AG, MacCormick AD. Weight Regain Following Sleeve Gastrectomy-a Systematic Review. Obesity Surgery. 2016;**26**:1326-1334

[4] Noel P, Nedelcu M, Eddbali I, Manos T, Gagner M. What are the long-term results 8 years after sleeve gastrectomy? Surg Obes Relat Dis Off J Am Soc Bariatr Surg. 2017;**13**:1110-1115

[5] Sjöström L. Review of the key results from the Swedish Obese Subjects (SOS) trial - a prospective controlled intervention study of bariatric surgery. Journal of Internal Medicine. 2013;**273**:219-234

[6] Freire RH, Borges MC, Alvarez-Leite JI, Toulson Davisson Correia MI. Food quality, physical activity, and nutritional follow-up as determinant of weight regain after Roux-en-Y gastric bypass. Nutr Burbank Los Angel Cty Calif. 2012;**28**:53-58

[7] Karmali S, Brar B, Shi X, Sharma AM, de Gara C, Birch DW. Weight recidivism post-bariatric surgery: a systematic review. Obesity Surgery. 2013;**23**:1922-1933

[8] Nedelcu M, Khwaja HA, Rogula TG. Weight regain after bariatric surgery-how should it be defined? Surg Obes Relat Dis Off J Am Soc Bariatr Surg. 2016;**12**:1129-1130

[9] King WC, Hinerman AS, Belle SH, Wahed AS, Courcoulas AP. Comparison of the Performance of Common Measures of Weight Regain After Bariatric Surgery for Association With Clinical Outcomes. Journal of the American Medical Association. 2018;**320**:1560-1569

[10] Lauti M, Lemanu D, Zeng ISL, Su'a B, Hill AG, MacCormick AD. Definition determines weight regain outcomes after sleeve gastrectomy. Surg Obes Relat Dis Off J Am Soc Bariatr Surg. 2017;**13:1123**-1129

[11] Carmeli I, Golomb I, Sadot E, Kashtan H, Keidar A. Laparoscopic conversion of sleeve gastrectomy to a biliopancreatic diversion with duodenal switch or a Roux-en-Y gastric bypass due to weight loss failure: our algorithm. Surg Obes Relat Dis Off J Am Soc Bariatr Surg. 2015;**11:79**-85

[12] Brethauer SA, Aminian A, Romero-Talamás H, et al. Can diabetes be surgically cured? Long-term metabolic effects of bariatric surgery in obese patients with type 2 diabetes mellitus. Annals of Surgery. 2013;**258**:628-636 discussion 636-637

[13] Liu SY-W, Wong SK-H, Lam CC-H, Yung MY, Kong AP-S, Ng EK-W. Long-term Results on Weight Loss and Diabetes Remission after Laparoscopic Sleeve Gastrectomy for A Morbidly Obese Chinese Population. Obesity Surgery. 2015;**25**:1901-1908

[14] Homan J, Betzel B, Aarts EO, van Laarhoven KJHM, Janssen IMC, Berends FJ. Secondary surgery after sleeve gastrectomy: Roux-en-Y gastric bypass or biliopancreatic diversion with duodenal switch. Surg Obes

Relat Dis Off J Am Soc Bariatr Surg. 2015;**11**:771-777

[15] Obeidat F, Shanti H, Mismar A, Albsoul N, Al-Qudah M. The Magnitude of Antral Resection in Laparoscopic Sleeve Gastrectomy and its Relationship to Excess Weight Loss. Obesity Surgery. 2015;**25:1928**-1932

[16] Bohdjalian A, Langer FB, Shakeri-Leidenmühler S, et al. Sleeve gastrectomy as sole and definitive bariatric procedure: 5-year results for weight loss and ghrelin. Obesity Surgery. 2010;**20:535**-540

[17] Jiménez A, Casamitjana R, Flores L, et al. Long-term effects of sleeve gastrectomy and Roux-en-Y gastric bypass surgery on type 2 diabetes mellitus in morbidly obese subjects. Annals of Surgery. 2012;**256**:1023-1029

[18] Angrisani L, Santonicola A, Iovino P, Formisano G, Buchwald H, Scopinaro N. Bariatric Surgery Worldwide 2013. Obesity Surgery. 2015;**25**:1822-1832

[19] Voorwinde V, Steenhuis IHM, Janssen IMC, Monpellier VM, van Stralen MM. Definitions of Long-Term Weight Regain and Their Associations with Clinical Outcomes. Obesity Surgery. 2020;**30**:527-536

[20] Amundsen T, Strømmen M, Martins C. Suboptimal Weight Loss and Weight Regain after Gastric Bypass Surgery-Postoperative Status of Energy Intake, Eating Behavior, Physical Activity, and Psychometrics. Obesity Surgery. 2017;**27**:1316-1323

[21] Abdallah E, El Nakeeb A, Youssef T, et al. Impact of extent of antral resection on surgical outcomes of sleeve gastrectomy for morbid obesity (a prospective randomized study). Obesity Surgery. 2014;**24**:1587-1594

[22] Courcoulas AP, King WC, Belle SH, et al. Seven-Year Weight Trajectories and Health Outcomes in the Longitudinal Assessment of Bariatric Surgery (LABS) Study. JAMA Surgery. 2018;**153**:427-434

[23] Braghetto I, Csendes A, Lanzarini E, Papapietro K, Cárcamo C, Molina JC. Is laparoscopic sleeve gastrectomy an acceptable primary bariatric procedure in obese patients? Early and 5-year postoperative results. Surgical Laparoscopy, Endoscopy & Percutaneous Techniques. 2012;**22**:479-486

[24] Shantavasinkul PC, Omotosho P, Corsino L, Portenier D, Torquati A. Predictors of weight regain in patients who underwent Roux-en-Y gastric bypass surgery. Surg Obes Relat Dis Off J Am Soc Bariatr Surg. 2016;**12**:1640-1645

[25] Baig SJ, Priya P, Mahawar KK, Shah S. Indian Bariatric Surgery Outcome Reporting (IBSOR) Group. Weight Regain After Bariatric Surgery-A Multicentre Study of 9617 Patients from Indian Bariatric Surgery Outcome Reporting Group. Obesity Surgery. 2019;**29**:1583-1592

[26] Kushner RF, Sorensen KW. Prevention of Weight Regain Following Bariatric Surgery. Current Obesity Reports. 2015;**4**:198-206

[27] Sundbom M, Holdstock C, Engström BE, Karlsson FA. Early changes in ghrelin following Roux-en-Y gastric bypass: influence of vagal nerve functionality? Obesity Surgery. 2007;**17**:304-310

[28] Tamboli RA, Breitman I, Marks-Shulman PA, et al. Early weight regain after gastric bypass does not affect insulin sensitivity but is associated with higher ghrelin levels. Obes Silver Spring Md. 2014;**22**:1617-1622

[29] Youssef A, Emmanuel J, Karra E, et al. Differential effects of laparoscopic sleeve gastrectomy and laparoscopic

gastric bypass on appetite, circulating acyl-ghrelin, peptide YY3-36 and active GLP-1 levels in non-diabetic humans. Obesity Surgery. 2014;**24**:241-252

[30] Santo MA, Riccioppo D, Pajecki D, et al. Weight Regain After Gastric Bypass: Influence of Gut Hormones. Obesity Surgery. 2016;**26**:919-925

[31] Sumithran P, Prendergast LA, Delbridge E, et al. Long-term persistence of hormonal adaptations to weight loss. The New England Journal of Medicine. 2011;**365**:1597-1604

[32] Meguid MM, Glade MJ, Middleton FA. Weight regain after Roux-en-Y: a significant 20% complication related to PYY. Nutr Burbank Los Angel Cty Calif. 2008;**24**:832-842

[33] Zalesin KC, Franklin BA, Miller WM, et al. Preventing Weight Regain After Bariatric Surgery: An Overview of Lifestyle and Psychosocial Modulators. Am J Lifestyle Med. SAGE Publications. 2010;**4**:113-120

[34] Rusch MD, Andris D. Maladaptive eating patterns after weight-loss surgery. Nutr Clin Pract Off Publ Am Soc Parenter Enter Nutr. 2007;**22**:41-49

[35] El Ansari W, El-Ansari K. Missing Something? Comparisons of Effectiveness and Outcomes of Bariatric Surgery Procedures and Their Preferred Reporting: Refining the Evidence Base. Obesity Surgery. 2020;**30**:3167-3177

[36] Saunders R. "Grazing": a high-risk behavior. Obesity Surgery. 2004;**14**:98-102

[37] Colles SL, Dixon JB, O'Brien PE. Grazing and loss of control related to eating: two high-risk factors following bariatric surgery. Obes Silver Spring Md. 2008;**16**:615-622

[38] Magro DO, Geloneze B, Delfini R, Pareja BC, Callejas F, Pareja JC. Long-term weight regain after gastric bypass: a 5-year prospective study. Obesity Surgery. 2008;**18**:648-651

[39] Rosenberger PH, Henderson KE, White MA, Masheb RM, Grilo CM. Physical activity in gastric bypass patients: associations with weight loss and psychosocial functioning at 12-month follow-up. Obesity Surgery. 2011;**21**:1564-1569

[40] Livhits M, Mercado C, Yermilov I, et al. Exercise following bariatric surgery: systematic review. Obesity Surgery. 2010;**20**:657-665

[41] Bond DS, Thomas JG, Unick JL, Raynor HA, Vithiananthan S, Wing RR. Self-reported and objectively measured sedentary behavior in bariatric surgery candidates. Surg Obes Relat Dis Off J Am Soc Bariatr Surg. 2013;**9**:123-128

[42] Sarwer DB, Wadden TA, Moore RH, et al. Preoperative eating behavior, postoperative dietary adherence, and weight loss after gastric bypass surgery. Surgery for Obesity and Related Diseases. 2008;**4**:640-646

[43] Rutledge T, Groesz LM, Savu M. Psychiatric factors and weight loss patterns following gastric bypass surgery in a veteran population. Obesity Surgery. 2011;**21**:29-35

[44] Sheets CS, Peat CM, Berg KC, et al. Post-operative psychosocial predictors of outcome in bariatric surgery. Obesity Surgery. 2015;**25**:330-345

[45] Mitchell JE, Christian NJ, Flum DR, et al. Postoperative Behavioral Variables and Weight Change 3 Years After Bariatric Surgery. JAMA Surgery. 2016;**151**:752-757

[46] Kofman MD, Lent MR, Swencionis C. Maladaptive eating patterns, quality of life, and weight

outcomes following gastric bypass: results of an Internet survey. Obes Silver Spring Md. 2010;**18**:1938-1943

[47] Freire CC, Zanella MT, Segal A, Arasaki CH, Matos MIR, Carneiro G. Associations between binge eating, depressive symptoms and anxiety and weight regain after Roux-en-Y gastric bypass surgery. Eat Weight Disord EWD. 2020; Jan 2. doi: 10.1007/s40519-019-00839-w. Online ahead of print.

[48] Kalarchian MA, Marcus MD, Wilson GT, Labouvie EW, Brolin RE, LaMarca LB. Binge eating among gastric bypass patients at long-term follow-up. Obesity Surgery. 2002;**12**:270-275

[49] Eid I, Birch DW, Sharma AM, Sherman V, Karmali S. Complications associated with adjustable gastric banding for morbid obesity: a surgeon's guides. Can J Surg J Can Chir. 2011;**54**:61-66

[50] Lanthaler M, Strasser S, Aigner F, Margreiter R, Nehoda H. Weight loss and quality of life after gastric band removal or deflation. Obesity Surgery. 2009;**19**:1401-1408

[51] Stroh C, Köckerling F, Volker L, et al. Results of More Than 11,800 Sleeve Gastrectomies: Data Analysis of the German Bariatric Surgery Registry. Annals of Surgery. 2016;**263**:949-955

[52] Kuzmak null, Burak null. Pouch Enlargement: Myth or Reality? Impressions from Serial Upper Gastrointestinal Series in Silicone Gastric Banding Patients. Obes Surg. 1993;**3**:57-62.

[53] Weiner RA, Weiner S, Pomhoff I, Jacobi C, Makarewicz W, Weigand G. Laparoscopic sleeve gastrectomy--influence of sleeve size and resected gastric volume. Obesity Surgery. 2007;**17**:1297-1305

[54] Braghetto I, Cortes C, Herquiñigo D, et al. Evaluation of the radiological gastric capacity and evolution of the BMI 2-3 years after sleeve gastrectomy. Obesity Surgery. 2009;**19**:1262-1269

[55] Noel P, Nedelcu M, Nocca D, et al. Revised sleeve gastrectomy: another option for weight loss failure after sleeve gastrectomy. Surgical Endoscopy. 2014;**28**:1096-1102

[56] Iannelli A, Schneck AS, Noel P, Ben Amor I, Krawczykowski D, Gugenheim J. Re-sleeve gastrectomy for failed laparoscopic sleeve gastrectomy: a feasibility study. Obesity Surgery. 2011;**21**:832-835

[57] Yimcharoen P, Heneghan HM, Singh M, et al. Endoscopic findings and outcomes of revisional procedures for patients with weight recidivism after gastric bypass. Surgical Endoscopy. 2011;**25**:3345-3352

[58] Heneghan HM, Yimcharoen P, Brethauer SA, Kroh M, Chand B. Influence of pouch and stoma size on weight loss after gastric bypass. Surg Obes Relat Dis Off J Am Soc Bariatr Surg. 2012;**8**:408-415

[59] Catalano MF, Rudic G, Anderson AJ, Chua TY. Weight gain after bariatric surgery as a result of a large gastric stoma: endotherapy with sodium morrhuate may prevent the need for surgical revision. Gastrointestinal Endoscopy. 2007;**66**:240-245

[60] Cucchi SG, Pories WJ, MacDonald KG, Morgan EJ. Gastrogastric fistulas. A complication of divided gastric bypass surgery. Annals of Surgery. 1995;**221**:387-391

[61] Filho AJB, Kondo W, Nassif LS, Garcia MJ, Tirapelle R de A, Dotti CM. Gastrogastric fistula: a possible complication of Roux-en-Y gastric bypass. JSLS. 2006;10:**326**-31.

[62] Al-Khyatt W, Ryall R, Leeder P, Ahmed J, Awad S. Predictors of Inadequate Weight Loss After Laparoscopic Gastric Bypass for Morbid Obesity. Obesity Surgery. 2017;**27**:1446-1452

[63] Paul L, van der Heiden C, Hoek HW. Cognitive behavioral therapy and predictors of weight loss in bariatric surgery patients. Current Opinion in Psychiatry. 2017;**30**:474-479

[64] Melton GB, Steele KE, Schweitzer MA, Lidor AO, Magnuson TH. Suboptimal weight loss after gastric bypass surgery: correlation of demographics, comorbidities, and insurance status with outcomes. J Gastrointest Surg Off J Soc Surg Aliment Tract. 2008;**12**:250-255

[65] Odom J, Zalesin KC, Washington TL, et al. Behavioral predictors of weight regain after bariatric surgery. Obesity Surgery. 2010;**20**:349-356

[66] Livhits M, Mercado C, Yermilov I, et al. Preoperative predictors of weight loss following bariatric surgery: systematic review. Obesity Surgery. 2012;**22**:70-89

[67] Ochner CN, Jochner MCE, Caruso EA, Teixeira J, Xavier P-SF. Effect of preoperative body mass index on weight loss after obesity surgery. Surg Obes Relat Dis Off J Am Soc Bariatr Surg. 2013;**9**:423-427

[68] Csendes A, Burgos AM, Martinez G, Figueroa M, Castillo J, Díaz JC. Loss and Regain of Weight After Laparoscopic Sleeve Gastrectomy According to Preoperative BMI : Late Results of a Prospective Study (78-138 months) with 93% of Follow-Up. Obesity Surgery. 2018;**28**:3424-3430

[69] Marek RJ, Ben-Porath YS, Dulmen MHM van, Ashton K, Heinberg LJ. Using the presurgical psychological evaluation to predict 5-year weight loss outcomes in bariatric surgery patients. Surg Obes Relat Dis Off J Am Soc Bariatr Surg. 2017;**13**:514-521.

[70] Capoccia D, Guida A, Coccia F, et al. Weight Regain and Diabetes Evolution After Sleeve Gastrectomy: a Cohort Study with over 5 Years of Follow-Up. Obesity Surgery. 2020;**30**:**1046**-1051

[71] Sarwer DB, Cohn NI, Gibbons LM, et al. Psychiatric diagnoses and psychiatric treatment among bariatric surgery candidates. Obesity Surgery. 2004;**14**:1148-1156

[72] McGrice M, Don PK. Interventions to improve long-term weight loss in patients following bariatric surgery: challenges and solutions. Diabetes Metab Syndr Obes Targets Ther. 2015;**8**:263-274

[73] Swenson BR, Saalwachter Schulman A, Edwards MJ, Gross MP, Hedrick TL, Weltman AL, et al. The effect of a low-carbohydrate, high-protein diet on post laparoscopic gastric bypass weight loss: a prospective randomized trial. The Journal of Surgical Research. 2007;**142**:308-313

[74] Marc-Hernández A, Ruiz-Tovar J, Aracil A, Guillén S, Moya-Ramón M. Effects of a High-Intensity Exercise Program on Weight Regain and Cardio-metabolic Profile after 3 Years of Bariatric Surgery: A Randomized Trial. Sci Rep [Internet]. 2020 [cited 2020 Aug 29];10. A.

[75] Thompson CC, Slattery J, Bundga ME, Lautz DB. Peroral endoscopic reduction of dilated gastrojejunal anastomosis after Roux-en-Y gastric bypass: a possible new option for patients with weight regain. Surgical Endoscopy. 2006;**20**:1744-1748

[76] Velapati SR, Shah M, Kuchkuntla AR, et al. Weight Regain

After Bariatric Surgery: Prevalence, Etiology, and Treatment. Curr Nutr Rep. 2018;**7**:329-334

[77] Kalarchian MA, Marcus MD, Courcoulas AP, Cheng Y, Levine MD, Josbeno D. Optimizing long-term weight control after bariatric surgery: a pilot study. Surg Obes Relat Dis Off J Am Soc Bariatr Surg. 2012;**8**:710-715

[78] Sarwer DB, Dilks RJ, West-Smith L. Dietary intake and eating behavior after bariatric surgery: threats to weight loss maintenance and strategies for success. Surg Obes Relat Dis Off J Am Soc Bariatr Surg. 2011;**7**:644-651

[79] Himes SM, Grothe KB, Clark MM, Swain JM, Collazo-Clavell ML, Sarr MG. Stop regain: a pilot psychological intervention for bariatric patients experiencing weight regain. Obesity Surgery. 2015;**25**:922-927

[80] Bradley LE, Forman EM, Kerrigan SG, Butryn ML, Herbert JD, Sarwer DB. A Pilot Study of an Acceptance-Based Behavioral Intervention for Weight Regain After Bariatric Surgery. Obesity Surgery. 2016;**26**:2433-2441

[81] Bradley LE, Forman EM, Kerrigan SG, et al. Project HELP: a Remotely Delivered Behavioral Intervention for Weight Regain after Bariatric Surgery. Obesity Surgery. 2017;**27**:586-598

[82] Lopes Gomes D, Moehlecke M, Lopes da Silva FB, Dutra ES, D'Agord Schaan B, Baiocchi de Carvalho KM. Whey Protein Supplementation Enhances Body Fat and Weight Loss in Women Long After Bariatric Surgery: a Randomized Controlled Trial. Obes Surg. 2017;**27**:424-31.

[83] Apovian CM, Aronne LJ, Bessesen DH, et al. Pharmacological Management of Obesity: An Endocrine Society Clinical Practice Guideline. J Clin Endocrinol Metab. Oxford Academic. 2015;**100**:342-362

[84] Tak YJ, Lee SY. Anti-Obesity Drugs: Long-Term Efficacy and Safety: An Updated Review. World J Mens Health. 2020; Mar 9. doi: 10.5534/wjmh.200010. Online ahead of print.

[85] Stanford FC, Alfaris N, Gomez G, et al. The utility of weight loss medications after bariatric surgery for weight regain or inadequate weight loss: A multi-center study. Surg Obes Relat Dis Off J Am Soc Bariatr Surg. 2017;**13**:491-500

[86] Istfan NW, Anderson WA, Hess DT, Yu L, Carmine B, Apovian CM. The Mitigating Effect of Phentermine and Topiramate on Weight Regain After Roux-en-Y Gastric Bypass Surgery. Obes Silver Spring Md. 2020;**28**:1023-1030

[87] Toth AT, Gomez G, Shukla AP, et al. Weight Loss Medications in Young Adults after Bariatric Surgery for Weight Regain or Inadequate Weight Loss: A Multi-Center Study. Child Basel Switz. 2018;**5**

[88] Schwartz J, Chaudhry UI, Suzo A, et al. Pharmacotherapy in Conjunction with a Diet and Exercise Program for the Treatment of Weight Recidivism or Weight Loss Plateau Post-bariatric Surgery: a Retrospective Review. Obesity Surgery. 2016;**26**:452-458

[89] C Sudlow A, W le Roux C, J Pournaras D. Review of Advances in Anti-obesity Pharmacotherapy: Implications for a Multimodal Treatment Approach with Metabolic Surgery. Obesity Surgery 2019;29:4095-104.

[90] Wharton S, Kuk JL, Luszczynski M, Kamran E, Christensen RAG. Liraglutide 3.0 mg for the management of insufficient weight loss or excessive weight regain

post-bariatric surgery. Clin Obes. 2019;**9**:e12323.

[91] Callahan ZM, Su B, Kuchta K, Linn J, Carbray J, Ujiki M. Five-year results of endoscopic gastrojejunostomy revision (transoral outlet reduction) for weight gain after gastric bypass. Surgical Endoscopy. 2020;**34**:2164-2171

[92] Parmar CD, Gan J, Stier C, Dong Z, Chiappetta S, El-Kadre L, et al. One Anastomosis/Mini Gastric Bypass (OAGB-MGB) as revisional bariatric surgery after failed primary adjustable gastric band (LAGB) and sleeve gastrectomy (SG): A systematic review of 1075 patients. Int J Surg Lond Engl. 2020;**81**:32-38

[93] Pearlstein S, Sabrudin SA, Shayesteh A, Tecce ER, Roslin M. Outcomes After Laparoscopic Conversion of Failed Adjustable Gastric Banding (LAGB) to Laparoscopic Sleeve Gastrectomy (LSG) or Single Anastomosis Duodenal Switch (SADS). Obesity Surgery. 2019;**29**:1726-1733

[94] Wu C, Wang F-G, Yan W-M, Yan M, Song M-M. Clinical Outcomes of Sleeve Gastrectomy Versus Roux-En-Y Gastric Bypass After Failed Adjustable Gastric Banding. Obesity Surgery. 2019;**29**:3252-3263

[95] Chiappetta S, Stier C, Scheffel O, Squillante S, Weiner RA. Mini/One Anastomosis Gastric Bypass Versus Roux-en-Y Gastric Bypass as a Second Step Procedure After Sleeve Gastrectomy-a Retrospective Cohort Study. Obesity Surgery. 2019;**29**:819-827

[96] Kraljević M, Süsstrunk J, Köstler T, Lazaridis II, Zingg U, Delko T. Short or Long Biliopancreatic Limb Bypass as a Secondary Procedure After Failed Laparoscopic Sleeve Gastrectomy. Obes Surg. 2020; Jul 23. doi: 10.1007/s11695-020-04868-8. Online ahead of print.

[97] Brown WA, Ooi G, Higa K, Himpens J, Torres A, IFSO-appointed task force reviewing the literature on SADI-S/OADS. Single Anastomosis Duodenal-Ileal Bypass with Sleeve Gastrectomy/One Anastomosis Duodenal Switch (SADI-S/OADS) IFSO Position Statement. Obes Surg. 2018;**28**:1207-16.

[98] Zaveri H, Surve A, Cottam D, et al. A Multi-institutional Study on the Mid-Term Outcomes of Single Anastomosis Duodeno-Ileal Bypass as a Surgical Revision Option After Sleeve Gastrectomy. Obesity Surgery. 2019;**29**:3165-3173

[99] Kraljević M, Köstler T, Süsstrunk J, Lazaridis II, Taheri A, Zingg U, et al. Revisional Surgery for Insufficient Loss or Regain of Weight After Roux-en-Y Gastric Bypass: Biliopancreatic Limb Length Matters. Obesity Surgery. 2020;**30**:804-811

Chapter 9

From Prehab to Rehab: The Functional Restoration of a Bariatric Individual

Anwar Suhaimi and Brenda Saria Yuliawiratman

Abstract

The bariatric population presents at a greater risk for functional decline with increasing weight and advancing age. This can be prevented at various time points through multidisciplinary rehabilitation interventions in a multitude of different settings to accommodate the severity of an individuals' disability and to target different functional goals. Bariatric rehabilitation is a multipronged approach that addresses the ongoing functional impairment, medical comorbidities, hospital-related deconditioning and prevents future cardiovascular and musculoskeletal complications from progressing. The emerging concept of utilising rehabilitation interventions and goal-centric approach as means to reduce post-operative complications and enhance surgical outcomes is also discussed. Pragmatic approaches to post-surgical bariatric rehabilitation are discussed highlighting the multi-faceted rehabilitation concerns to achieve optimal functionality in the face of a chronic medical condition.

Keywords: bariatrics, rehabilitation, recovery of function, exercise, behaviour modification

1. Introduction

Bariatric individuals not only present with specific medical complications and more prevalent risk factors for cardiovascular disease (CVD) and musculoskeletal (MSK) conditions, this population also has significantly greater potential for functional decline. Graded increase in activities of daily living (ADL) limitation was observed with increasing body weight [1]. Rehabilitation medicine approach to address the needs of a bariatric individual encompasses both ends of the management spectrum: to restore and prevent further deterioration of physical function associated or aggravated with excess body weight; as well as to enhance post-operative results with a sustainable weight management strategy.

The rehabilitation medicine approach to function can be viewed from The International Classification of Functioning, Disability and Health (ICF) concept to better understand the interactive nature of a chronic health condition such as obesity and formulate a rehabilitation plan to address physical, psychological and socio-environmental barriers to bariatric-related disability [2, 3] (**Table 1**). Individualisation of care from all disciplines involved in the bariatric population

Domains affected	Descriptors
Body function	Energy and drive function
	Weight maintenance functions
Activities and participation	Handling stress and other psychological demands
	Walking
	Moving around
	Looking after one's health
Environmental factors	Products of substances for personal consumption
	Immediate family

Table 1.
Brief ICF Core set for Obesity [3].

to produce long-term sustainable results can also be deduced by understanding the dynamics of a disease process through this concept. We shall discuss the approaches to a bariatric evaluation, rehabilitation intervention and functional outcome in two parts with special focus on prehabilitation and peri-operative rehabilitation.

2. Addressing bariatric functional limitations

Obesity affects physical, biopsychosocial aspects of an individual's health and function. The complex nature may require rehabilitation interventions to be carried out in various settings to accommodate for different functional goals and engaging a multidisciplinary rehabilitation team to tap into different expertise to achieve the desired functional milestones. The bariatric individual presents with unique challenges to the treating team in both functional limitations and the approaches that can be employed to address these impairments and prevent further functional deterioration. The ICF highlights the domains that are affected by excessive weight: pain, cutaneous sensation, neuromusculoskeletal issues and movement difficulties as well skin issues due to difficulty in reaching during cleaning and toileting are the most commonly impaired function and complications leading to limitation in general tasks, mobility and poorer quality of life [1]. Concurrent presence of medical comorbidities can add up to tip the individual into compromised functional independence [1]. Common comorbidities related to obesity such as osteoarthritis of the weight bearing joints and cardiopulmonary conditions impacts severely on an individual's functional reserves. Thus, the goal for bariatric rehabilitation program should include assisting the attainment of optimal weight reduction; to address current and potential medical complications especially metabolic syndrome, CVD and MSK conditions; to address functional limitations resulting from physical disabilities and improve quality of life through improving functional independence, self-confidence and empowering self-management.

Severe obesity with multiple comorbidities requires admission to medical facilities structurally adequate to assist in supporting and assisting individuals with excess body mass to transfer and mobilise with the use of bariatric- safe lifting devices, mobility equipment and transfer aids. Ideally these rehabilitation facilities are linked to a bariatric- dedicated medical and surgical specialities [4].

The bariatric patients frequently develop medical complications that may run a protracted course [5]. Common medical complications readily noted at admission include:

- Skin excoriations, rashes or ulcers in deep tissue folds with possibility of fungal infections.

- Edema or fluid retention and venous congestion that causes feeling of limb heaviness or leading to diaphoresis-fluid leakage that renders the skin sensitive to shear forces, skin tears and infection.

- Diabetes and respiratory problems including obesity hypoventilation syndrome or obstructive sleep apnoea.

These complications may indicate specialised nursing care or aids to protect during mobilisation. It may also preclude the use of some rehabilitation modalities i.e. hydrotherapy and priorities needs to be given to address medical conditions that delays resumption of weight bearing or therapeutic standing.

Hospitalisation-related complications that tend to occur are mainly as a result of prolonged recumbency, also known as deconditioning. While deconditioning is not exclusive to bariatric population, its effects are more pronounced as bariatric individuals face challenges for immediate resumption of upright posture especially those who were admitted acutely for medical complications such as cardiopulmonary emergencies, following falls or exacerbation of musculoskeletal conditions leading to pain on weight bearing. Deconditioning can affect both physical and psychological domains as prolonged bed rest affects nearly all body systems. Specific to bariatric population these complications may entail a prolonged stay and protracted course of recovery:

- Cardiovascular system: orthostatic hypotension and reduced exercise tolerance contributed by decreased cardiac output and resting tachycardia affecting sitting up, standing, transfers and physical activity participation.

- Pulmonary system: orthostatic pneumonia or atelectasis resulting in hypoxemia and reduced tolerance to physical activity may complicate obesity hypoventilation syndrome or sleep apnoea.

- Haematological system: deep venous thrombosis and pulmonary embolism may occur despite no lower limb neurological deficit as abdominal mass may compress on lower limb circulation and altered blood viscosity.

- Musculoskeletal system: muscle atrophy causing weakness; leading to longer periods of non-weight bearing and increasing the risk of osteoporosis, joint stiffness and worsening posture. Especially of concern is weakness of extensor muscles needed to assume or assist to an upright position.

- Gastrointestinal: constipation from lack of upright posture often complicate prescription diet plans due to the bloating sensation, abdominal discomfort and possibility of spurious diarrhoea complicating personal hygiene due to poor access to the perineal region combined with postural stasis that predisposes to the development of pressure ulcers.

- Endocrine: impaired insulin response with hyperglycemia; gastrostasis leading to sensation of nausea and oesophageal reflux symptoms.

The result impacts on a bariatric individual's functional reserves in terms of muscle power, balance, and coordination, jeopardising functional performance and results in the development of psychological sequelae as a direct result of deconditioning or from the loss of function it entails. Confusion and disorientation are part of the deconditioning constellation seen earlier on the bedrest period which can culminate in clinically significant anxiety and depression once the impact of functional loss sets in as self-care, leisure activities and gainful employment becomes challenging. Reconditioning as a rehabilitation goal will be discussed further in the prehabilitation section. Given the prospect of functional deterioration that can occur at an accelerated rate in the bariatric population due to inherent difficulties in mobilisation, special attention should be given to addressing factors that negate upright sitting and to promote lower limb weight bearing in cases that permit them as soon as possible. These include identifying at risk bariatric individuals with hip and knee replacements, paralysis, amputations, contractures, osteoporosis, respiratory and cardiac conditions, and skin conditions such as pressure ulcers. Availability of bariatric mobility aids such as hoists, tilt tables, chairs or wheelchairs and walking aids greatly assist in preventing the ill effects on deconditioning and translates to better cost-efficiency to prevent such deleterious complications rather than treatment of the aforementioned complications.

Various models of bariatric rehabilitation exists to generally addresses 5 key factors: knowledge to empower action, goal-setting and self-care; beliefs surrounding causes and solutions to obesity; behavioural adaptation focusing on diet and physical activity, psychological coping strategies and adjustments of physical activity to include exercise, current functional capacity and that expected after bariatric surgery. A holistic model such as bio-psycho-social model explained via ICF helps to provide a multi-dimensional framework to evaluate the needs, identify the barriers and provide intervention or solutions to improve independence. Selection of the model to address such an individualistic experience such as function is paramount as the different considerations of the desired rehabilitation goals and outcomes of interest are given priority by different models [6]. The lack of obesity-specific outcome measures to quantify physical impairments and ADL limitations prevents stratification of bariatric individuals based on the magnitude of disability [7]. This is useful to establish as a threshold value for inpatient rehabilitation admission, and serves as an objective severity identification tool that impacts on the decision of appropriate rehabilitation setting and chart progress during rehabilitation. An example of such tool is the Obesity-related Disability Test (TSD.OC) developed by Donini et al. that aims to evaluate pertinent obesity- specific functional dimensions [8]. The main targets for bariatric rehabilitation are the cardiorespiratory, musculoskeletal and multi-systemic effects of deconditioning as described above. Strategies that reduce pain, increases strength and mobility as well as optimise functions can be delivered in various settings depending on the severity of obesity-induced disability. Inpatient rehabilitation facility offers an opportunity for more intensive rehabilitation input and caters well to bariatric clients admitted acutely for MSK or CVD that often runs a prolonged hospital stay and poorer functional recovery if left without rehabilitation input. The goals of inpatient rehabilitation are focused on attaining maximal functional independence for safe home discharge through improvements in strength, balance, and endurance coupled with initiation of CVD risk factor control and body weight reduction through dietary and physical activity prescription. An outpatient program may provide significant functional improvements in clients who can access both the centres and their lodging with appropriate means of transportation between them. This is attained by promoting increased pain-free joint range of motion, increasing muscle strength and cardiopulmonary endurance during functional activities. Concurrent efforts to optimise CVD risk factor and improve lean-to-fat mass ratio are also continued in the outpatient setting through education and individualised counselling on dietary and physical activity plan to maximise functional capacity despite excessive weight. Capodaglio et al. conducted a prospective 4-week inpatient bariatric rehabilitation with orthopaedic conditions consisting of strengthening and aerobic exercises adapted to the patient's mobility; caloric restriction and nutritional education with psychological counselling [7]. The results exemplified that mild and severely disabled bariatric individuals with orthopaedic comorbidities can significantly experience functional improvements independent of the weight loss sustained; with the higher BMI and younger individuals showing the most functional gains. Similarly, Hanapi et al. employed an approach based on the cardiac rehabilitation model and resources for inpatient bariatric clients with CVD risk factors and orthopaedic comorbidities [9]. Employing adapted physical activity and exercise prescription, dietary modification, provision of psychological and social support, their approach successfully addressed weight, cardiometabolic profile optimisation prior to bariatric surgical intervention and conferring postoperative improvement in mood, dependency level, perceived physical and mental health during the postoperative phase with sustained functional capacity, endurance and quality of life up to 3 months post operatively.

Admission planning for an inpatient rehabilitation stay is crucial to ensure logistic requirements, staffing ratio, bariatric-compliant equipment, administrative support and a mobilisation plan is developed as part of a function-centric rehabilitation plan. By definition, bariatric individuals include individuals whose weight exceeds or appears to exceed the identified safe working loads for equipment, lacks mobility or presents with challenges in manual handling [10, 11]. Moving and handling of bariatric clients can accentuate the risks of musculoskeletal injuries and excessive spinal loading in health care workers. Planning of staff and equipment reduces the risks associated with the care of bariatric patients. Safety of patients and health care workers can be enhanced by developing a movement and handling plan as each bariatric admission often presents with unique issues that require problem solving and an understanding of equipment or patient transfer procedures. Involvement of occupational health and safety representatives as well as risk reduction efforts can minimise unplanned situations that may differ between patients due to individuals' risks, goals and resources available. Every aspect of patient- HCW interaction should be therapeutic from rehabilitation perspective including communication. Open discussion on equipment use and transfer techniques can lead the way to more serious discussions on dietary habits, adapting lifestyles and long-term functional goals. Education on the importance of physical activity and dietary management to aid weight loss and maintain functional independence helps boost motivation and compliance [9]. Discharge planning should include not just physical preparation of the destination. Consideration should be given to post-rehabilitation functional limitations that may require physical help or adaptive equipment as functional goals attainment may require repeated cycles of rehabilitation. Potential home modifications and long-term plans for adapted physical activity, dietary maintenance, psychological support, surveillance for relapses and complications as well as plans for higher functions such as return to work and driving should be discussed with the patients and their social support.

Outpatient bariatric rehabilitation continues the inpatient gains made with focus on long-term prevention of function and weight- gain relapse. The common impairments addressed are osteoarticular pain especially of the lower back and knees as well as joint malalignment. The effects of excessive weight on systemic inflammation, joint compression and premature degenerative disease of the joint can be offset by the role of adapted physical activity which is more pronounced in this setting to maintain compliance to caloric expenditure, CVD prevention and positive psychosocial reinforcement. A combination of both aerobic, resistance and flexibility exercises adapted to individual MSK conditions working on large muscle groups alongside dietary modification has led to improvement in CV biomarkers, fat loss and skeletal muscle gains conferring enhanced functional improvements in programs that include resistance exercises [12, 13]. In comparison to diet modification intervention alone, multimodal exercises program combined with diet interventions conferred lean mass sparing effect [14]. This is also evident in a systematic review of sarcopenic obesity treatment whereby excess fat mass and reduced lean mass impairs physical performance in which weight loss attained through exercise in combination with dietary intervention is the best treatment strategy that improves metabolic consequences of excess fat mass while preserving lean muscle mass and promotes functional recovery [15]. Aerobic exercises for caloric expenditure, reducing joint pain and controlling weight which is a risk factor of osteoarthritis as well as resistance exercise for strengthening of the joint supporting musculature and cartilage health reduces obesity-related joint conditions [16, 17]. As the client returns to the community, psychological support to sustain weight loss motivation and purpose as well as addressing stigma associated with excessive weight is equally important to ensure sustained functional and weight loss gains are maintained. Chronic pain and its effect on gait, psychical activity, participation and quality of life also needs to be addressed.

In conclusion, bariatric rehabilitation addresses common medical comorbidities and obesity related MSK complications through multimodal rehabilitative and allied health interventions, including prescription exercises and diet modification to increase cardiopulmonary endurance and caloric expenditure while minimising fear of movement and joint pain. This in turn leads to progressive body weight reduction and improved comorbidities profile leading to better body composition and physical function capacity.

3. Prehabilitation: Maximising post-operative outcomes

Bariatric individuals often present with medical comorbidities arising from obesity-related changes or complications sustained from hospitalisation- related bedrest for acute medical crises. Functional impairments evident pre-operatively should be addressed to improve postoperative results and functional independence. The concept of deconditioning is discussed above- the bariatric individual runs a higher risk of developing deconditioning due to delayed weight bearing or resumption of an upright position. This is often multifactorial: common patient related factors such as sarcopenia, kinesiophobia, osteoarticular joint pain and exertional dyspnoea; logistic issues i.e. lack bariatric-safe equipment or staffs' lack of ergonomic awareness are among easily amenable factors [18]. Deconditioning impacts the geriatric age group more [19]. Adapted exercises have been successful to prevent multisystem deconditioning from zero-gravity environment or from prolonged bed rest [20, 21]. Hanapi et al. demonstrated a 6-weeks bariatric surgery prehabilitation [9] consisting of patient education and prescription of therapeutic exercises, dietary modification and nutritional-behavioural counselling, the use of technological advancement to facilitate early non-weight bearing aerobic and resistance exercises that had successfully prepared the bariatric patients for the demands of the surgery as well as facilitated early post-operative mobilisation that has been purported to reduce post-surgical morbidity [22, 23]. This model adapted the principles of cardiac rehabilitation in formulating the evaluation, intervention and outcomes including risk-stratifying the bariatric surgery candidates for cardiovascular risk during exercise participation, quantifying exercise capacity for exercise prescription and addressing CVD risk factors that can complicate anaesthetic and post-operative care. Priorities were given to utilising adapted physical activity and early mobilisation to translate cardiorespiratory and musculoskeletal reserve improvements into functional mobility and independence in basic activities of daily living. This model along with other bio-psycho-social approaches have shown positive impact on long term functional capacity, endurance, dietary habits, weight loss and quality of life up between 3 to 12-month post-surgery [24].

In the management of a complex, chronic condition such as obesity a multidisciplinary approach has consistently shown the best outcomes [25]. This approach however must be integrated into individual clinical complexity of each individual bariatric patient. An approach that entail evaluation with the intent to individualise treatment plan utilising multimodal treatment strategies i.e. diet, physical activity and functional rehabilitation, educational therapy, cognitive-behaviour therapy, drug therapy, and bariatric surgery will most likely ensure quality of weight loss, addressing the medical and psychiatric comorbidities together, psychosocial problems and physical disability [26]. Older bariatric patients may face a more challenging rehabilitation course due to age-related changes such as sarcopenia, muscular fatty infiltration which leads to strength reduction and diminishing exercise capacity; as well as external factors such as increased inertia from excessive mass causing imbalance, longer exposure to effects of obesity causing pronounced musculoskeletal degeneration and pain as well as more damage in the peripheral tissues [7]. Sarcopenic obesity in advanced age contributes to more dependence in ADL [27]. Muscular and mobility deterioration in combination contributes to exacerbate physiological changes associated with ageing. Thus, identification of such patients earlier prior to surgery is paramount to ensure successful outcomes following bariatric surgery.

The economics of bariatric rehabilitation can be seen from 2 angles- in respect to functional restoration and from a long-term preventive viewpoint. Bariatric individuals who have undergone rehabilitation have shown functional improvement independent of the amount of weight lost, with more pronounced improvement in function observed in the severely disabled individuals [7]. This translates to earlier weight bearing, resumption of mobility and independence in self-care which in turns minimises the risk post-operative complications. Alongside improvement in muscular strength and lean mass, individuals who have undergone rehabilitation also had controlled CVD risk profiles, joint pain and reduced sedentary time conferring protection to future CVD in this high-risk group. However, to truly understand the cost–benefit effect of bariatric rehabilitation, long term outcomes expressed in multiple domains of function are needed to allow better understanding of the effect of different rehab interventions, optimal intensity and duration to therapeutic effect.

Capacity building in an organisation that caters for bariatric rehabilitation is essential to reduce personal risks to patients and staff as well as minimise disruption of bariatric rehabilitation services. This includes developing a bariatric rehabilitation pathway, continuous staff education and training and an audit of the outcomes from the pathway. A bariatric rehabilitation pathway details the appropriate facilities, staff and equipment are available at each stage of the bariatric individuals' rehabilitation process from admission to outpatient facilities. Although this may incur short term increase in expenditure, the long term return of investment can be quantified through better morbidity and mortality reduction of the bariatric population regardless of conservative or surgical management approach chosen to suit individual medical and functional needs.

4. Rehabilitation following bariatric surgery

Formulation of an individually-tailored rehabilitation program based on each bariatric patients' clinical complexity should be the priority to holistically manage such clients using a multidisciplinary team approach. Multidisciplinary teams offer the best post-operative outcomes [28], addressing quality of weight loss, medical and psychiatric comorbidities, psychosocial problems and physical disability [29]. To ensure a smooth transition from prehabilitation through postoperative rehabilitation, the physical, biopsychosocial model continues to be relevant and emphasis should be placed on preventing surgical-related complications, secondary prevention of CVD, addressing bariatric-related disabilities, psychological and socio-environmental barriers, enhancing physical function through adapted physical activities, education on nutritional management as well as implementation of sustainable weight management strategies.

The post-bariatric surgery management will require coordinated care from a multidisciplinary team of healthcare providers starting from immediate post-op followed by long-term management. The integration of several medical specialties including clinical nutrition, endocrinology, psychiatry [1], rehabilitation medicine, as well as allied health professionals including physiotherapy, occupational therapy, and nursing should be included as part of the core management team. Each team member should provide detailed assessment of impairments, outline prevention strategies and provide solutions for disease management alongside implementation of a functional restoration program. A functional restoration program post-operatively should aim to not only achieve marked weight loss, but also prevention of weight regain, progression of obesity-associated comorbidities, restoration of physical functioning and increase health-related quality of life.

A post-op functional restoration program can be broadly grouped into two categories:

1. Medical

   i. Nutritional management

   ii. Weight management

   iii. Comorbidities

2. Rehabilitation

   i. Physical activity and exercise training

   ii. Psychosocial

4.1 Medical

4.1.1 Nutritional management

The goal of weight loss procedures in general is to either reduce the amount of consumed calories (restrictive) per day or to alter the absorption of the fat (malabsorption) in the food one consumes. For restrictive procedures such as vertical banded gastroplasty (VBG) or laparoscopic adjustable gastric banding (LAGB), that has no malabsorption effect, the volume of food intake will be reduced overall, hence, some nutritional deficiencies may occur. Malabsorptive surgeries such as or biliopancreatic diversion (BPD), gastric sleeve (GS) or Roux-en-Y gastric bypass (RYGB) causes alterations in the intestinal tract and creates challenges in maintaining healthy levels of nutrients including proteins, vitamins and minerals as well as reduction in the absorption of calcium and iron [30].

Management of these potential nutritional deficiencies is therefore paramount for patients undergoing bariatric surgery and strategies should be employed to compensate for food reduction or food intolerance to reduce the risk for clinically important nutritional deficiencies. Signs and symptoms of protein deficiency such as hair loss, fatigue and leg swelling should be monitored. Heber et al. recommended the nutritional management should include: an average of 60 – 120 g of protein daily in all patients to maintain a lean body mass during the weight loss and for the long term to prevent protein malnutrition and its effects, and this is especially important in those treated with malabsorptive procedures to prevent protein malnutrition and its effects [28].

Long-term vitamin and mineral supplementation is recommended in all patients undergoing bariatric surgery with those who have had malabsorptive procedures requiring potentially more extensive replacement therapy to prevent nutritional deficiencies [28]. Specific signs and symptoms of common vitamin and mineral deficiencies include bone pain (calcium), fatigue (iron, vitamin B12), brittle nails (zinc), poor wound healing (vitamin E), easy bruising (vitamin K), numbness and tingling in the hands and feet (vitamin B1). Deficiencies in fat-soluble vitamins A, D, E and K is expected therefore, it is essential for patients to take specially formulated vitamins (A, D, E, and K in water-soluble form). B-complex vitamins, iron, and calcium must also be supplemented at higher than daily recommended levels, because of the impact of the gastric bypass procedure on their absorption. Due to the body's limited ability to a absorb calcium postoperatively and the acidic environment needed for absorption, a citrated form of calcium is recommended and taken in amounts that meet or exceed daily recommended levels [30]. For maximal absorption, elemental calcium supplements should be taken in divided doses not to exceed 500 mg, three times daily [30]. Iron deficiency is also very common after malabsorptive procedures and iron-fortified foods such as leafy greens, legumes, seafood, iron-fortified grains, red meat and poultry should be consumed on a regular basis. Routine laboratory testing of the iron stores postoperatively may be required with iron supplementation either orally or parenterally administered accordingly by the healthcare provider.

Dumping syndrome may occur as a result of malabsorptive procedures such as RYGB where the food content empties into the small intestine faster than usual. Patients may experience symptoms such as abdominal cramping, nausea and vomiting due to the small intestine being unable to absorb the nutrients from food that have not been fully digested in the stomach. Reactive hypoglycaemia may also occur due to the large surge of insulin after "dumping". Dietary changes is the mainstay of treatment for dumping syndrome. Avoidance of simple carbohydrates such as white flour and sugar, consumption of more complex carbohydrates such as whole grain and sources of protein such as fish, meat, beans, legumes and soy are recommended. Frequent loose stools is also a potential side-effect of malabsorptive procedures. It is critical that patients stay adequately hydrated to reduce the risk of dehydration. Lack of mobility may also predispose patients with regular soiling of the perineum to skin pathologies including development of pressure areas. Nutritional education is vital to the success of the surgery and prevention of complications. Regular follow-up and periodic monitoring of nutritional deficiencies postoperatively will be required for detection and correction. Lifelong supplementation of daily mineral, multivitamin and micronutrients must be considered.

4.1.2 Weight management

Following weight loss surgery, patients may lose weight fairly rapidly at first, and then as time passes the weight loss becomes more gradual. Commonly, weight will stabilise at about 18 months after RYGB [30]. During these 18 months, weight loss can be erratic with alternating periods of significant weight loss followed by a plateau. Other than the loss of fat mass, there are many other factors that may contribute to the fluctuations in weight loss during the initial phase. This includes variations in water weight which is dependent upon the individuals' hydration status, contents of the gastrointestinal tract, gain of muscle mass, or menstrual cycles [30].

Sustainable weight loss strategies should include tailored exercise programs with monitoring of the exercise frequency and intensity to boost metabolic rate for a more rapid weight loss. A generic exercise program with lack of progressive targeted goals may lead to weight loss plateaus. Increase in physical activity and strength training will cause slower weight loss as the fat is replaced by muscle mass, which are denser tissues. This should not be perceived as a deterrent, but rather a positive trend that will lead to a leaner frame and stronger body. The recommended nutritional plan should be adhered to diligently to ensure adequate nutrition and muscle mass is maintained. Most weight regain or plateaus in weight loss boils down to eating habits. It is recommended that a patient eat several small meals a day with the ultimate goal of eating a regular diet in smaller amounts. Binge eating, snacking or grazing should be avoided as the extra calories will add up to the weight gain.

Several anatomic factors may influence weight loss, and this include the size of the gastric pouch which may change over time with the RYGB. As it enlarges over time, it will accommodate larger meals, causing a reduction in weight loss. Anostomotic dilatation between the stomach pouch and the intestine may also occur and this allows quicker emptying of the pouch, reducing its effect on satiety and potential weight loss [30]. This is also the underlying reason why one should not drink during meals after gastric bypass as it will result in a more rapid transition of solid food from the gastric pouch, eliminating the effect on satiety resulting in ingestion of larger portions. The resultant change in anatomic structure after malabsorptive procedures such as the RYGB also alters the absorption of food with higher absorption of fats, thus reducing the benefit of the surgery [30]. Eating small meals high in protein may help mitigate this effect.

Plateaus and fluctuations in weight loss are to be expected throughout various phases post-surgery. Constant reassurance, providing patient education on the expected outcomes and exploring together the underlying causes of weight plateaus can increase understanding, avoid miscommunication, avert patient depression or frustration with the surgery. A regular exercise regimen and adherence to correct eating behaviour and nutritional intake may lead to greater outcome and a more sustainable long-term weight loss.

4.1.3 Comorbidities

Frequently, patients undergoing bariatric surgery have associated comorbidities including Type 2 Diabetes Mellitus, cardiovascular disease, lipid abnormalities, fatty liver, degenerative joint disease, hypertension, gastroesophageal reflux disease, and obstructive sleep apnea with considerable impact on disability and quality of life. To reduce the likelihood of weight regain and to ensure that comorbid conditions are adequately managed, all patients should receive careful medical follow-up postoperatively. Monitoring postoperative glycaemic control should consist of achieving glycated HBA1c of 7% or less with fasting blood glucose no greater than 110 mg/dl and postprandial glucose no greater than 180 mg/dl [28]. Lipid abnormalities should be monitored and treated with lipid-lowering therapy that remain above desired goals should be continued. However due to the dramatic reductions in lipid levels, the doses of lipid-lowering drugs should be periodically evaluated [28]. Ideally, a multidisciplinary team should be in place before the operation is performed. The bariatric surgeon should be part of this comprehensive team that provides pre- and postoperative care. The inclusion of other medical specialties in the team including endocrinologists, gastroenterologists and rehabilitation physicians allow a more holistic approach for the treatment of patients with multiple comorbidities and associated impairments and disabilities.

4.2 Rehabilitation

4.2.1 Physical activity and exercise

Surgery-induced weight loss by itself was associated with a series of beneficial health effects, including increased objectively measured habitual physical activity and cardiorespiratory fitness [29]. Using a cardiac rehabilitation model is effective to cause significant improvement in bariatric individuals' cardio-metabolic profile [31]. Hanapi et al. demonstrates the application of cardiac rehabilitation principle for post-bariatric surgery patients which include risk stratification through the use of submaximal exercise stress testing to objectively quantify the patient's cardiovascular capacity for exercise participation, subsequent exercise prescription based on the individuals' physical impairments and cardiovascular functioning, lifestyle modification to manage cardiovascular risk factors and translating the gains of cardiorespiratory and musculoskeletal fitness into more functional activities [9].

Postoperative exercise is imperative and remains the most important factor that can help a patient achieve long-standing and successful weight loss. Exercises can begin as early as day one postoperatively and short term and long term goals should be set early on and revised as activity and exercise capacity increases. The exercise program should incorporate muscle strengthening, physical endurance or aerobic exercises to improve cardiorespiratory fitness, balance training, functional mobility, musculoskeletal reconditioning, joint protection as well activity of daily living (ADL) training, tailored individually within the limit of patients' cardiovascular capacity.

To sustain weight loss, effective behaviour changes towards increasing energy expenditure through occupational, leisure time and planned physical activity needs to occur alongside dietary management [32]. Physical activity can be incorporated to daily activities which helps with caloric expenditure or decreasing the amount of sitting time or sedentary leisure activities. Education on the importance of physical activities to aid weight loss and maintain functional independence helps boost motivation and compliance. This ultimately affects their level of independence, quality of life and self-efficacy [9].

In addition to loss of fat mass, there are other numerous benefits to exercise. These benefits include prevention of loss of muscle mass when losing weight rapidly after surgery, and improved overall weight loss. Exercise may also reduce a person's appetite, increases immunity and reduces fatigue which may lead to improved self-confidence, and overall improved sense of well-being.

4.2.2 Psychosocial

A substantial number of patients experience poor long-term outcomes following bariatric surgery which may be contributed by difficulty in making and sustaining changes in dietary intake and physical activity as well as post-surgery binge eating, which has also been associated with poorer weight outcomes [33]. A thorough pre-operative assessment to evaluate patients' understanding of the disease condition, identifying any misconceptions, assessing readiness and commitment to undergo a radical change in lifestyle and behaviour modification, as well identifying issues that may pose as barriers may be the key to a successful and sustainable weight management postoperatively. Sheets et al. recommend that preoperative assessment should include identifying patients strengths and weaknesses, educating patients thoroughly about postoperative changes including dietary intake and physical activity, coaching on lifestyle change strategies as well as offering specific recommendations to address any areas of concern [34]. The period post bariatric surgery is still a vulnerable time for most individuals as the reality sinks in as adjustment of behaviours and new habits take place. The need for continuous care and screening of psychosocial issues throughout both pre-and postoperative periods cannot be undermined. Screening for aberrant eating behaviours and depressive symptoms should be assessed whilst administering interventions to address emotional and psychological issues, behavioural modification strategies, increase compliance, and provide support [34]. It is the responsibility of each team member to detect or identify the presence of any psychological issues, and administer interventions through early referral to mental health professionals to improve outcomes of these individuals.

Author details

Anwar Suhaimi[1]* and Brenda Saria Yuliawiratman[2]

1 Department of Rehabilitation Medicine, Faculty of Medicine, University of Malaya, Kuala Lumpur, Malaysia

2 Rehabilitation Medicine Unit, Department of Orthopedics and Traumatology, Faculty of Medicine, The National University of Malaysia, Kuala Lumpur, Malaysia

*Address all correspondence to: anwar@ummc.edu.my

References

[1] Capodaglio P et al. *Disability in obesity with comorbidities. A perspective from the PRM societies*. European Journal of Physical and Rehabilitation Medicine. 2014;**50**(2):129-132

[2] Robinson KT, Butler J. *Understanding the causal factors of obesity using the international classification of functioning, disability and health*. Disability and Rehabilitation. 2011;**33**(8):643-651

[3] Projects ICSICF. *Core Set for*. Obesity. 2017 Available from: https://www.icf-research-branch.org/icf-core-sets-projects2/cardiovascular-and-respiratory-conditions/icf-core-set-for-obesity

[4] *Disabling Obesity: From Determinants to Health Care Models*. 2013.

[5] Seida JC et al. *Hospital rehabilitation for patients with obesity: A scoping review*. Disability and Rehabilitation. 2018;**40**(2):125-134

[6] Forhan M. *An analysis of disability models and the application of the ICF to obesity*. Disability and Rehabilitation. 2009;**31**(16):1382-1388

[7] P C, VK H, J L. *Effectiveness of multidisciplinary inpatient and outpatient rehabilitation on functional outcomes in obese patients with orthopedic comorbidities*. In: *Disabling Obesity*, P.C.e. al. Berlin Heidelberg: Springer-Verlag; 2013. pp. 107-124

[8] Donini L, Brunani A. A.S.e. al, *Assessing disability in morbidly obese individuals: the Italian society of obesity test for obesity-related disabilities*. Disability and Rehabilitation. 2010:1-10

[9] Hanapi NHM et al. *Optimising the bariatric Patients' outcome through cardiac rehabilitation approach*. Obesity Surgery. 2018;**28**(7):2130-2134

[10] *Information Sheet – Moving and Handling the Bariatric Patient*, Q. Health, Editor. 2010. p. 48.

[11] Robertson H. *Managing Obese and Bariatric Patients in an Acute Hospital Setting*. Sydney, Australia: *The importance of establishing a bariatric working party*. in *Biennial Conference of the Association for Manual Handling of People*; 2010

[12] Davidson L. And R.H.K.K.e. al, *Effects of exercise modality on insulin resistance and functional limitation in older adults: a randomized controlled trial*. Archives of Internal Medicine. 2009;**16**(2):122-131

[13] Villareal D, Chode S. And N.P.e. al, *Weight loss, exercise, or both and physical function in obese older adults*. The New England Journal of Medicine. 2011;**364**(13):1218-1229

[14] Frimel T, Sinacore D, Villareal D. *Exercise attenuates the weight-loss-induced reduction in muscle mass in frail obese older adults*. Medicine and Science in Sports and Exercise. 2008;**40**(7):1213-1219

[15] Poggiogalle E et al. *Treatment of body composition changes in obese and overweight older adults: Insight into the phenotype of sarcopenic obesity*. Endocrine. 2014;**47**(3):699-716

[16] Suri P, Morgenroth D, Hunter D. *Epidemiology of osteoarthritis and associated comorbidities*. PMR. 2012;**4**:S10-S19

[17] Vincent H, Bourguignon C, Vincent K. *Resistance training lowers exercise-induced oxidative stress and homocysteine levels in overweight and obese older adults*. Obesity. 2006;**14**(11):1921-1930

[18] Kortebein P. *Rehabilitation for hospital-associated deconditioning*.

American Journal of Physical Medicine & Rehabilitation. 2009;**88**:66-77

[19] H, H. and R. L. *Hospital-associated deconditioning and dysfunction*. Journal of the American Geriatrics Society. 1991;**39**(2):220-222

[20] Ploutz-Snyder LL et al. *Exercise training mitigates multisystem deconditioning during bed rest*. Medicine and Science in Sports and Exercise. 2018;**50**(9):1920-1928

[21] Maggioni MA et al. *High-intensity exercise mitigates cardiovascular deconditioning during long-duration bed rest*. Frontiers in Physiology. 2018;**9**:1553

[22] Zhang, L., et al., *Early mobilization of critically ill patients in the intensive care unit: A systematic review and meta-analysis.* PLOS ONE, 2019. **14**(10): p. e0223185.

[23] de Almeida EPM et al. *Early mobilization programme improves functional capacity after major abdominal cancer surgery: A randomized controlled trial*. BJA: British Journal of Anaesthesia. 2017;**119**(5):900-907

[24] Jassil, F.C., et al., *Feasibility and Impact of a Combined Supervised Exercise and Nutritional-Behavioral Intervention following Bariatric Surgery: A Pilot Study.* J Obes, 2015. **2015**: p. 693829.

[25] Capodaglio P et al. *Rehabilitation in obesity with comorbidities: A consensus document from experts of the Italian Society of Physical and Rehabilitation Medicine (SIMFER), the Italian Society of Obesity (SIO) and the Italian Society of Eating Disorders (SISDCA)*. Eating and Weight Disorders. 2014;**19**(3):383-386

[26] Donini LM et al. *From simplicity towards complexity: The Italian multidimensional approach to obesity*. Eating and Weight Disorders. 2014;**19**(3):387-394

[27] Jensen G, Hsiao P. *Obesity in older adults: Relationship to functional limitation*. Current Opinion in Clinical Nutrition and Metabolic Care. 2010;**13**(46-51)

[28] Heber D. And e. al, *Endocrine and nutritional management of the post-bariatric surgery patient: an Endocrine Society Clinical Practice Guideline*. The Journal of Clinical Endocrinology and Metabolism. 2010;**95**(11):4823-4843

[29] Oppert J. And e. al., *Resistance Training and Protein Supplementation Increase Strength After Bariatric Surgery: A Randomized Controlled Trial*. Obesity. 2018;**26**(11):1709-1720

[30] Surgery, A.S.f.M.a.B. *Postoperative Concerns*. 2008; Available from: https://asmbs.org/resources/bariatric-surgery-postoperative-concerns.

[31] Rodriguez-Escudero JP. And e. al, *Effect of a lifestyle therapy program using cardiac rehabilitation resources on metabolic syndrome components*. Journal of Cardiopulmonary Rehabilitation and Prevention. 2013;**33**(6):360-370

[32] Ades PA, Savage PD, Harvey-Berino J. *The treatment of obesity in cardiac rehabilitation*. Journal of Cardiopulmonary Rehabilitation and Prevention. 2010;**30**(5):289-298

[33] Kalarchian M, Marcus M. *Psychosocial interventions pre and post bariatric surgery*. European Eating Disorders Review. 2015;**6**:457-462

[34] Sheets C. And e. al., *Post-operative psychosocial predictors of outcome in bariatric surgery*. Obesity Surgery. 2015;**25**(2):330-345